RACE HYGIENE AND NATIONAL EFFICIENCY

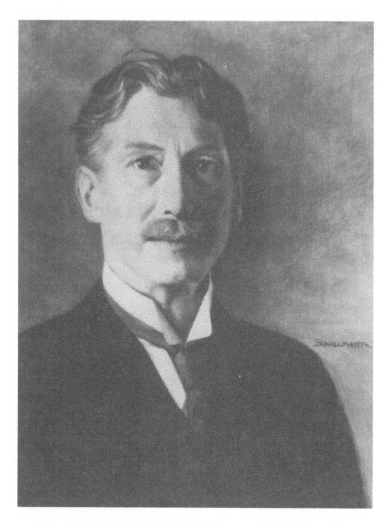

Portrait of Wilhelm Schallmayer in 1918.
Courtesy of his son, Fredrick Schallmayer.

RACE HYGIENE AND NATIONAL EFFICIENCY

The Eugenics of Wilhelm Schallmayer

SHEILA FAITH WEISS

UNIVERSITY OF CALIFORNIA PRESS
Berkeley   Los Angeles   London

Dedicated to my husband, Michael,
and to my mother and the memory
of my father, with love and gratitude

University of California Press
Berkeley and Los Angeles, California

University of California Press, Ltd.
London, England

Copyright © 1987 by The Regents of the University of California

Library of Congress Cataloging-in-Publication Data
Weiss, Sheila Faith.
    Race hygiene and national efficiency.
    Bibliography: p.
    Includes index.
    1. Schallmayer, Wilhelm, 1857 – 1919. 2. Heredity.
3. Eugenics. I. Title.
HM106.W45   1987   304.5   86-24895
ISBN 0-520-05823-2

1 2 3 4 5 6 7 8 9

CONTENTS

PREFACE

Two considerations spurred my initial interest in and subsequent investigation of the subject matter of this book: my desire for a dissertation topic that promised to bridge the gap between my two scholarly interests, history of biology and modern German history, and the lack of any study dealing specifically with the history of German eugenics. That I should have viewed German eugenics as an appropriate historical subject, given my interdisciplinary bias, is not particularly surprising. Puzzling, however, was the historiographical reticence surrounding the topic. Even when I first began to explore my dissertation project ten years ago, several books had already been published on the eugenics movements in Britain and the United States. Yet nothing existed for Germany comparable to Mark Haller's useful *Eugenics: Hereditarian Attitudes in American Thought*, or Geoffrey Searle's brief but insightful *Eugenics and Politics in Britain*, to name only two of the numerous books and articles dealing with Anglo-American eugenics. Only much later did I realize that the tendency to classify German eugenics simply as a part of the history of European racism, plus the taboo placed on the subject by the German medical establishment, explained why so little had been written on the subject. I too assumed that I would find in the German eugenics movement, and particularly in the writings of Germany's eugenicists, a mere biological legitimation of anti-Semitism. After all, I figured, what other purpose could eugenics in Germany have had if not to point out the racial inferiority of the Jews? That my first hunch was wrong makes the study that follows, if not less interesting than it might have been, at least, I hope, more provocative.

Most of the research for the dissertation from which the book originated was done in the Federal Republic of Germany and was financed by both a National Foundation Travel Grant, and a two-year predoctoral Fulbright scholarship. While in Germany the Fulbright-Kommission and the Deutscher Akademischer Austauschdienst each provided me with a badly needed Goethe Institute language course, for which I am deeply grateful. Both my research and well-being were promoted by the warm reception of the faculty and students of the Medizinhistorisches Institut of the Johannes Gutenberg-Universität in Mainz. In particular, I would like to thank the director of the Institute, Professor Dr. Gunter Mann, as well as Professor Dr. Werner Kümmel for giving me access to an excellent library, and providing me with an office and a stimulating intellectual environment during my two-year stay in Mainz. While in Germany I also profited from my discussions with Professor Dr. Hans Querner of the Institut für Geschichte der Medizin, Abteilung Geschichte der Biologie of the Ruprecht-Karl Universität in Heidelberg. For her friendship and her help in translating Schallmayer's letters I am indebted to Dr. Ingrid Schumacher. Lastly, I would like to thank Friedrich Schallmayer and Wilfrid Ploetz for the information they furnished me concerning their fathers. Friedrich Schallmayer also graciously provided me with the photograph of his father.

The following individuals deserve my special thanks for their valuable comments and criticisms during the dissertation stage of my project: Robert Kargon and Vernon Lidtke, both from The Johns Hopkins University; Pat Gossel and Tom Cornell, Rochester Institute of Technology; William Coleman, University of Wisconsin, Madison; Donna Haraway, University of California, Santa Cruz; W. R. Albury, University of New South Wales, Sydney, Australia; Mark Adams, University of Pennsylvania. I am especially grateful to my former adviser Owen Hannaway of The Johns Hopkins University for his numerous insightful suggestions and his insistence on clarity and precision in my work.

The revision of my dissertation manuscript was made possible in part by a Mellon Foundation research grant and release time awarded by the Faculty of Liberal Studies, Clarkson University, and a National Science Foundation Summer Scholar's Grant in 1984 for research in the German Democratic Republic and West Berlin. I would like to thank Professor Dr. Horst Franke and Dr. Erika Krauße, of the Ernst Haeckel-Haus in Jena for giving me access to correspondence pertaining to the Krupp competition as well as for their help in securing accommodations during my stay. While in West Berlin I was extremely fortunate to make the acquaintance of two of the most knowledgeable historians of German eugenics, Professor Dr. Gerhard Baader and Dr. Michael Hubenstorf, both of the Institut für Geschichte der Medizin of the Freie Universität. Not only did they make me aware of the extraordinarily large volume of German literature produced during the last five years dealing at least tangentially with the history of German eugenics but also helped me to place my own work in the broader context of the intellectually rich, if still largely taboo, topic of Nazi medicine. I have profited both personally and intellectually from our growing friendship. Finally, I would like to thank Jeff Johnson, Villanova University, for providing me with his notes from the Krupp Archive.

My list of acknowledgements would be incomplete without mentioning my debt to my mother, my late father, and above all, my husband, Michael Neufeld. Without the love and financial backing of my parents I most certainly would never have been able to attend college, let alone produce a scholarly book. Michael has helped me in more ways than can be easily stated. He not only provided me with ample emotional support but also acted as colleague, editor, typist, and proofreader—always putting my needs above his own. His love, patience, and devotion made the completion of this manuscript both possible and worthwhile.

INTRODUCTION

The statesman whose vision is not merely directed at momentary success and whose horizon has been broadened by the light of the theory of descent would recognize that the future of his nation is dependent on the *good management* of its reproductive [human] resources.

Wilhelm Schallmayer[1]

"Eugenics" is a political strategy denoting some sort of social control over reproduction. In the interest of "improving" the hereditary substrate of a given population, this supposed science seeks to regulate human procreation by encouraging the fecundity of the allegedly genetically superior groups in society and simultaneously discouraging and even prohibiting so-called inferior types from having children. The mere definition of the term, of course, does not account for a curious historical fact: the proliferation, beginning around the turn of the century, of eugenics movements in most Western and in several Far Eastern and Latin American countries.[2] Until recently, however, only Anglo-American eugenics has been the subject of serious scholarly investigation.[3] Indeed as a result of this historical preoccupation with the movements in Britain and the United States, Anglo-American developments have wittingly or unwittingly been used as a "standard" by which to judge and evaluate eugenics in other countries. To be sure, one always runs the risk of distorting the past by holding up any historical development in a particular nation or group of nations as a model for the assessment of similar developments elsewhere, and it is fortunate that scholars working on the history of the eugenics movements in France and Brazil, for example, have finally begun to correct this problem.[4] Yet anyone attempting to explore eugenics in Germany is beset by still another, far more difficult obstacle: preconceived notions regarding the aims, and, to a lesser extent, the "uniqueness" of the German movement. Ask most lay people and even many historians what comes to mind when the words "German eugenics" or "German race hygiene"[5] are mentioned and the answer is always the same: the Holocaust. Virtually everyone assumes that, in Germany, eugenics was limited to the breeding of a better "Aryan race." Whereas in Britain, so the story goes, eugenics was primarily concerned with *class*, its German counterpart was preoccupied with *race*.[6] In the German context, the connection between the "scientific" regulation of human reproduction and the "final solution" appears both obvious and straightforward.

Since the 1960s this "gut reaction" has been strongly reinforced in numerous publications dealing with the history of German or European racism. Often treating German eugenics in a very cursory manner, these works—insofar as they place race hygiene within the framework of racist, *völkisch*, and anti-Semitic ideologies—have obscured not only the context in which German eugenics developed (as part of a larger international movement) but also the legacy of the early movement for both post-1933 race hygiene and Nazi racial policy.[7] Happily, this state of affairs has improved. No longer content with histories of German eugenics that treat it as part of some other larger story, scholars on both sides of the Atlantic have begun to study race hygiene as a subject in its own right. The resulting newer literature, much of which is in German or is relatively obscure, has done an important service by deemphasizing the connection between race hygiene and Aryan race theory.[8] Yet several recent excellent studies on specific German eugenic practices and institutions notwithstanding,[9] no one has either attempted to provide a viable account for the appearance of race hygiene, or adequately explained its logic and rationale. Concentrating by and large on the more immediately significant Weimar and Nazi periods, these historians have all but ignored the formative early years of the movement—presumedly on the grounds that it does not shed much light on the subsequent development of race hygiene. Hence, despite the existence of these newer studies, important questions remain unasked, let alone answered. What, for example, is race hygiene in Germany fundamentally about? How and under what circumstances did it get started? And finally, what, if anything, is the connection between Wilhelmine eugenics, race hygiene under the swastika, and the bestial racial policies undertaken by the Third Reich?

This study seeks to answer these questions by examining the writings of the physician Wilhelm Schallmayer (1857–1919) who, along with Alfred Ploetz (1860–1940), founded German eugenics. Although Schallmayer was not particularly active in the German movement's organizational development, his numerous books and articles gave Wilhelmine eugenics its theoretical foundation. His short 1891 treatise, *Über die drohende körperliche Entartung der Kulturmenschheit und die Verstaatlichung des ärztlichen Standes* (Concerning the Imminent Physical Degeneration of Civilized Humanity and the Nationalization of the Medical Profession) was the first eugenics tract published in Germany.[10] Here we find, some thirteen years prior to the beginning of the German eugenics movement, a clearly articulated strategy for saving Western civilization as a whole, and Germany in particular, from the peril of "degeneration."

The Krupp competition of 1900 and the subsequent publication, in 1903, of his award-winning second book, *Vererbung und Auslese im Lebenslauf der Völker* (Heredity and Selection in the

Life History of Nations), brought Schallmayer and the cause of
eugenics to the attention of large segments of Germany's educated middle classes. In fact, the publicity given to his views as a
result of the competition was in no small measure responsible
for the organizational and institutional growth of the German
eugenics movement. Passing through three revised editions,
Schallmayer's *Vererbung und Auslese* remained the standard eugenics textbook throughout the first generation of the movement. The book not only discussed critical theoretical issues underlying eugenics but also spelled out a practical eugenics
program, large portions of which were adopted by the Deutsche
Gesellschaft für Rassenhygiene (German Society for Race
Hygiene).

Schallmayer's undoubted importance is not, however, the
primary reason for focusing on him. He was the first person
to clearly articulate the technocratic/managerial logic behind
German eugenic thought, indeed behind eugenic thought in
general: the idea that power or "national efficiency" is essentially a problem in the rational management of population.[11] A
close examination of Schallmayer's writings reveals that German
race hygiene was a sometimes conscious, oftentimes unconscious strategy to boost national efficiency (which also meant, in
the German context, cultural productivity) through a kind of
rational management or managerial control over the reproductive capacities of various groups and classes. Such a rational
administration of Germany's stock of human resources,
Schallmayer believed, would ensure the necessary level of hereditary fitness thought to be a prerequisite for the long-term survival of Germany and Western Europe and the allegedly superior
cultural traditions they embodied.

For Schallmayer the rational management of population
meant limiting the reproduction of the "unfit." Schallmayer's
equation of hereditary fitness with social productivity, and to a
large degree social class, led him to focus his attention on Germany's least productive citizens—criminals, alcoholics, the in-

sane, the feeble-minded—whose numbers, as a result of their increased visibility in industrial society, appeared to be rapidly growing. These asocial individuals (one might argue that they represented a subproletarian class) became, in biomedical terminology, Schallmayer's "hereditary degenerates,"—the unfit.

But limiting the reproduction of the "unfit" was only half the story. Schallmayer recognized that he would have to find some way to encourage the reproduction of the "fit" if Germany was to hold her own among the "civilized" nations of the world. As a result of late marriages, birth control, and excessive "egoism," Germany's biologically and socially most valuable citizens, the educated middle classes, seemed to be headed for gradual extinction. Unless someone could convince the "fittest" groups to make a statistically larger contribution to the biological endowment of the Reich, the nation of Goethe, Schiller, and Kant would fall prey to proletarian mediocrity—it would "degenerate." Thus Schallmayer proposed a rational administration of population as the only means of effectively redressing the growing imbalance between genetically inferior and superior material. "Rational selection"—to be encouraged by a combination of propaganda and, to a much lesser extent, legislation—was the best way to solve the so-called problem of degeneration.

In sum, Schallmayer's writings give us the opportunity to examine German race hygiene in the context of the social, political, and intellectual history of the Empire, and provide a valuable insight into the origins of race hygiene. An investigation of the works of Schallmayer also reveal their similarity to other non-German eugenics writings, especially to those of leading figures in Britain, and helps to undermine the assumption that German race hygiene was unique among eugenics movements. But most important, a study of Schallmayer's works unmasks race hygiene's underlying logic and rationale. This logic—the management of population as a means of boosting national efficiency—was not idiosyncratic: it was prevalent in the writings of virtually all German eugenicists throughout the history of the race hygiene movement. Indeed this logic formed the common bond which united those race hygienists who accepted ideologies of Aryan supremacy and those non-racist[12] eugenicists, like Schallmayer, who vehemently rejected them. As will become evident in the Epilogue, the ominous role of this logic for certain Nazi racial policies is unmistakable.

I

THE SOCIAL, PROFESSIONAL, AND INTELLECTUAL ORIGINS OF SCHALLMAYER'S EUGENICS

THE SOCIAL CONTEXT: INDUSTRIALIZATION AND THE "SOCIAL QUESTION"

During Schallmayer's lifetime Germany was transformed from an agricultural to an industrial society. Unlike Britain and France, where a similar transformation began earlier and extended over a longer period of time, German industrialization, to use Ralf Dahrendorf's well-known aphorism, "occurred late, quickly, and thoroughly."[1] After a slow beginning in the 1840s, the industrial revolution took off during the period 1850–1873. Spurred by the development of the textile industry; the extension of the German railroad network; and the rapid growth of the mining, steel, and machine industries, industrial capitalism quickly penetrated all sectors of the national economy. During the second phase, the so-called Great Depression (1873–1895), industrialization proceeded somewhat more slowly and severe recessions were frequent. Nevertheless, it was in this period that industry supplanted agriculture as the dominant form of production in the new Kaiserreich that was founded in 1871 after the defeat of France. Finally, in the third phase of German industrialization (1896–1913), huge industrial cartels appeared in heavy industry, and the chemical and electrical engineering industries grew to world stature. The rapid economic growth of this period soon brought the Reich to the position of third most important industrial power in the world, after the United States and Britain.[2]

Hand in hand with expeditious industrialization went accelerated urbanization. Beginning around mid-century and reaching its completion before 1910, the process of urban development transformed Germany from a predominantly rural society to a nation where over half the population dwelt in towns or cities.[3] At the time of unification just slightly more than one third of all Germans lived in towns with two thousand inhabitants or more; by 1910, 60 percent of all citizens could be found in towns of the same size. Moreover, whereas in 1871 only 4.8 percent of the population made their home in cities over a hundred thousand, in 1910, 21.3 percent of all inhabitants resided in such large urban centers.[4] This urbanization process that was inseparable from industrialization, inevitably altered the class structure of German society.

Industrialization and urbanization not only effected profound changes in the social and economic structure of Germany but also precipitated myriad serious social tensions and problems that, owing to the country's rigidly authoritarian political foundation, often threatened to upset the very stability of the young nation. The constitutional structure of the Kaiserreich as worked out by Bismarck guaranteed that Germany's preindustrial elites—the East Elbian Prussian landed aristocracy, the military, and high-ranking members of the bureaucracy—in collaboration with the new barons of industry would be able to successfully thwart all attempts at meaningful political participation by the rest of society. Parliament and universal male suffrage notwithstanding, neither the industrial and artisanal working classes nor large segments of the nonindustrial middle class were able to gain the upper hand in German politics. Through repression,

manipulation, compensation, and indoctrination, Germany's ruling elites sought both to contain the new forces of industrial
modernity and to placate those who felt uneasy in the new industrial order, without eliminating the social tensions of a political system both unable and unwilling to accept fundamental
change.[5]

Foremost among the problems afflicting the Reich as a result
of this combination of political immobility and rapid social
change was the rise of a radical labor movement. Born in the
1860s, the Social Democratic party (SPD) and its related trade
unions had by the turn of the century won the allegiance of the
majority of German industrial workers and had become the most
powerful force for social change in the country. Bismarck's attempt to crush the labor movement in its infancy through the
Anti-Socialist Laws (1878 – 1890) merely resulted in the adoption
of a more radical, Marxist position before the law was finally
repealed.[6] The growing number of strikes, lockouts, and other
forms of labor unrest, coupled with the increasing success of the
SPD at the polls, only served to exacerbate further the fear and
anxiety of many middle-class and upper-class Germans regarding the seemingly hostile, uncontrollable, and ever-increasing industrial proletariat.[7]

In addition to the labor movement, there was a whole series
of other, albeit less serious, social problems which were viewed
by Germany's *Bildungsbürgertum* (educated middle classes) as a
threat to the proper functioning of the state. One of the most
important of these was the increase in various types of criminal
activity. Although the common perception of a growing army of
criminals out to destroy the social fabric of society was undoubtedly an exaggeration, there was indeed a marked increase in
violent and nonviolent crime after 1880.[8] It is estimated that by
1898 over 1 percent of all Germans old enough to be convicted
possessed a criminal record.[9] Particularly alarming was the rapid
rise in criminal recidivism and juvenile delinquency. In Prussia
alone the number of "repeat offenders" more than doubled
between 1883 and 1901; during this same period the delin-

quency rate for minors increased by over one third.[10] This growth in criminal activity not only promoted a sense of uneasiness and fear among respectable, law-abiding Germans, but also drained the nation's treasury: in 1898 approximately one hundred million marks were spent to prosecute and detain the Reich's lawbreakers.[11]

No less anxiety-provoking for the self-righteous and order-loving Bildungsbürgertum was the increase in prostitution, alcohol consumption, and alcoholism. Though hardly a new vice, prostitution remained a relatively small-scale, inconspicuous phenomenon until the first phases of German industrialization.[12] Despite all attempts to contain and control it, prostitution reached what many observers considered to be epidemic proportions by the end of the nineteenth century. Estimates of the total number of prostitutes in the Reich for this period vary from one hundred to two hundred thousand.[13] Exacerbating the serious social and moral affront of prostitution were its medical consequences: widespread venereal disease.

During the industrial revolution Germany also experienced a sharp increase in the general level of alcohol consumption. Between 1850 and 1873, for example, the amount of hard liquor (measured in volume of pure alcohol) consumed per individual per year rose 44 percent; beer intake (measured in the same terms) increased a staggering 112 percent from 1850–1875.[14] A rise in the number of reported incidents of intoxication and alcoholism, especially among working-class drinkers, accompanied the growth of beer and schnapps consumption in this period. In the 1880s there were over eight thousand arrests per year for public drunkenness in Berlin alone.[15] Both press and pulpit discussed the mounting "alcohol problem" throughout the last decades of the nineteenth century, and concerned citizens began an open attack by creating several private, professional, and church-sponsored temperance organizations.[16]

Although not usually viewed as a social problem in the narrow sense of the term, Germany's insane and feeble-minded also became objects of both lay and professional (medical) attention during the Kaiserreich. Physicians and statisticians debated whether the rapid growth in the number of institutions for these "mental defectives" (as they were later called) testified to an absolute rise in the proportion of the number of insane and feeble-minded relative to the general population. Some were adamant in their belief that mental degeneration was on the rise.[17] Others, like Schallmayer, were less certain that the sharp increase in the number of patients detained and/or eventually treated in Germany's asylums constituted substantial proof that insanity was becoming more prevalent, and preferred to use statistics documenting a substantial rise in suicides—up 20 percent between 1881 and 1897—as evidence for an increase in the "mentally degenerate."[18] Whatever the reason for the large number of insane and retarded (an estimated 136,000 institutionalized individuals in 1901)[19] and whatever methods were used to demonstrate the growth of their ranks, they were undoubtedly perceived as a grave social and financial liability for the new Reich.

All these problems were viewed by many observant Bildungsbürger as a threat to a well-functioning German society. In fact, less than a year after Bismarck's political unification in 1871 academic social scientists and reform-minded religious leaders began what became a quite heated and protracted debate over the so-called *soziale Frage* (social question)—the social and political consequences of unbridled economic liberalism and industrialization.[20] Heavily influenced by cameralist traditions, the German historical school of economics, and philosophical idealism (Hegelianism), men like economists Adolf Wagner and Gustav Schmoller, and Lutheran minister Friedrich Naumann warned that the profits and power amassed by Germany's most recent special interest group—the industrialists—could continue to grow only at the expense of the commonweal. Manchesterism and rapid industrialization, according to these reformers, destroyed the traditional social and economic order,[21] leaving Germany with a hostile industrial proletariat and an increasing number of asocial individuals (the subproletariat). Only the state, as guardian of the common good, was in the position to solve the social question and reestablish the social harmony necessary to sustain a stable and prosperous *Kulturstaat*. As one author summarized Schmoller's perception of the problem:

> If we do not succeed in at least moderating the unresolved class conflict and the exploitation of the lower classes by the upper classes, the existing culture will go the way of earlier cultures—it will crumble—just as history has demonstrated on so many occasions.[22]

Germany's social scientists, civil servants, and middle-class intellectuals felt that the national interest compelled them to adopt some form of *Sozialpolitik* (social policy) to help redress the much discussed social question.

Of the numerous organizations formed to debate and propose solutions to the social question, none was more important than the Verein für Sozialpolitik (Society for Social Policy). Founded in 1872 by Wagner, Schmoller, and the economist Lujo Brentano, the Society reflected the anti-laissez faire biases of the reform-minded, academic social scientists who comprised the great majority of the association. Strongly anti-Marxist while at the same time embracing Marx's organicism[23] and social critique of capitalism, the members of the Society rejected the "peculiar utilitarian ethic of entrepreneurial individualism," and sought to prohibit "economic man" from "impos[ing] his preferences upon the rest of the nation."[24] Although individual members embraced different economic ideals (ranging from state socialism to a modified version of economic liberalism), all viewed economic activity as subservient to larger and more important cultural and political ends. Their position demanded that social reform be undertaken from the standpoint of the whole society, not any one particular class. Indeed, as Fritz Ringer has pointed out, the very term *Sozialpolitik* implied a "social or communal" approach to solving the social question, not an individualistic (or class-biased) one.[25] In reality, however, social policy was an attempt by a handful of academically trained middle-class intellectuals to integrate the industrial proletariat (and the asocial subproletariat) into German society with a minimal amount of damage to the political status quo. In the last analysis Sozialpolitik was a strategy to ensure the stability of the state by preempting a social revolution.

The extent to which middle-class intellectuals outside the Society shared this preoccupation with the soziale Frage can be gleaned by the rise of a number of reform-minded voluntary organizations. For example, the Deutscher Verein gegen den Mißbrauch geistiger Getränke (German Association for the Prevention of Alcohol Abuse), one of the most important of these middle-class associations, sought a solution to the social question by attacking the "drink question." Expressing the social activism of a broad cross section of the Bildungsbürgertum, the Association preached the gospel of temperance in order to create, among other things, an orderly, industrious working class and "a more harmonious and therefore more efficient industrial society."[26]

A preoccupation with the social question was not the only thing uniting Germany's educated middle classes. Although it would be an oversimplification to speak of a unified Bildungsbürgertum possessing a unitary political and social outlook, the social scientists, the temperance enthusiasts, and eugenicists such as Schallmayer did share a common if rather general set of assumptions about the nature of culture, society, and the state.[27] Perhaps most significant was the Bildungsbürger's veneration of Kultur. Feeling ill at ease in an industrial society increasingly dominated by two major classes, labor and capital, the Bildungsbürger took pride in his position as standard-bearer of German culture. For the educated middle-class German, the social prestige associated with a Gymnasium and university education (where culture was absorbed and transmitted) was far more important than the material wealth that served as a basis for Germany's new economic class.[28] Like the industrial middle class however, the Bildungsbürgertum grew more conservative as the rise of a radical working class appeared to threaten the very foundation of society. Social imperialism and social

Darwinism became increasingly appealing to educated middle-class Germans.[29] Moreover, true to the German statist tradition—a tradition that equated the interest of society with that of the state, and placed the well-being of the latter above everything else—the Bildungsbürger mocked the special interest group mentality of Germany's political parties, and longed for a leader above the parties who was capable of solving the Reich's most pressing social problems.[30]

As we will see, the Bildungsbürgertum's disgust with the parties, its statism, and its idealization of social harmony and stability were all reflected in Schallmayer's eugenics. Indeed, his eugenic strategy can be viewed as a new type of Sozialpolitik which mirrored both the prejudices and social concerns of his class. Like all educated middle-class Germans, Schallmayer was keenly aware of the profound social and economic changes which accompanied the industrial revolution, and was anything but oblivious to the serious social problems and tensions which plagued the Reich as a result. The increased visibility of a number of asocial, nonproductive types—an important, if not the most important component of the social question—was the problem which Schallmayer and other eugenicists set out to tackle by means of race hygiene.

PROFESSIONAL COMMITMENT:
THE GERMAN MEDICAL TRADITION

Attempts to effectively deal with the social question were not, of course, the monopoly of any one professional or occupational group. Most, if not all, university trained Germans acknowledged the existence of a problem and recognized that their own well-being demanded its speedy solution. However, the various occupational groups comprising the Bildungsbürgertum discussed and sought to remedy the problem differently—each according to a whole series of unarticulated and perhaps unperceived guidelines dictated by the social, political, and intellectual traditions of the particular profession in question. Schallmayer was a physician by training. As such, he not only shared the prejudices and posture of the Bildungsbürgertum as a whole but also inherited a well-defined set of assumptions about: (1) the social and political role of medical professionals in safeguarding the health of the nation, and (2) the hereditary nature of disease.

By and large late nineteenth- and early twentieth-century medical professionals shared the same socially conservative outlook as other educated middle-class Germans. Like other university trained individuals, they viewed themselves as part of the prestigious intellectual elite—an elite responsible, at least in their eyes, for the preeminence of German culture.[31] The physicians' social conservatism and sense of social superiority was further reinforced by the exclusiveness of the medical profession, and by the large number of professional organizations and associations to which the vast majority of practitioners belonged. The latter proved to be especially important in promoting an image of physicians as morally and intellectually superior beings who were "born into their profession." Germany's numerous medical associations also served to socialize physicians. Most of the organizations demanded that members adhere to social and ethical codes designed to dictate and regulate their conduct and worldview. Any affronts to the medical *Standesehre* (professional honor) were punished by medical review boards specifically created to ensure that doctors remain worthy of their noble occupation.[32]

Politically, physicians in Imperial Germany differed little from other Bildungsbürger. As was the case with the majority of educated middle-class Germans, medical doctors clung to a whole series of generally accepted, if not well-defined political attitudes such as nationalism, social Darwinist-inspired imperialism, and militarism.[33] Yet like most Bildungsbürger, German doctors professed to be apolitical. True to the statist tradition of German political theory, Germany's "apolitical" doctors revered the ideal of a conflict-free society where all groups and classes worked for the interest of the whole. For most, involvement in party politics was beneath their professional dignity. Political parties catered merely to special interests, it was believed; medicine and medical practitioners served the welfare of the entire nation![34]

The medical professionals' perception of themselves as custodians of national health, and hence national wealth and culture, dates at least as far back as the health reform movement during the Revolution of 1848–1849.[35] Taking their lead from the French public hygiene movement, medical men such as Rudolf Virchow and Salomon Neumann sought to demonstrate beyond doubt the causal relationship between poverty, squalor, and disease. Since health, according to Virchow and Neumann, was directly affected by adverse social factors such as poor diet, improper sanitary conditions, and a low standard of living, physicians were compelled to go beyond the traditional medical means of safeguarding the health and well-being of the community; they must work to improve the social conditions of their fellow countrymen and women.[36] For the reformers, such improvement implied far-reaching political and economic changes. Yet even in the short run much could be done to upgrade the health of the population by enacting a comprehensive public health program, then a radically new idea in the German states.

The public health program envisaged by the reformers and articulated in such documents as Neumann's draft for a Public Health Law[37] reflected the aspirations of numerous politically conscious physicians and large segments of the then-liberal Bildungsbürgertum. The health reformers' dream of a comprehensive public health program, like the liberals' dream of unification, remained just that.[38] Yet the reformers' perception of themselves as German patriots and civil servants, their belief in the efficacy of medicine as a means of solving social problems, and their demand that physicians play an active role in raising the level of health in society left a deep imprint on the minds of both contemporary and future medical professionals.[39]

Whatever the reformers thought of their contribution to the well-being of the nation, the prestige and social status enjoyed by physicians during the first half of the century was not particularly high.[40] Nor was the reactionary period of the 1850s and early 1860s a particularly advantageous time for physicians to further their professional aspirations. Many of the physicians' associations designed to give medical professionals control over their own affairs disappeared owing to disinterest.[41] The two decades following German unification in 1871, however, did witness a marked change of circumstances, especially for university-based medical researchers. The rise of scientific medicine—a development made possible by the maturation of such basic sciences as microscopic anatomy, physiology, and pathology in the laboratories of the reformed German universities—bestowed upon academic physicians, and the medical profession in general, an unprecedented level of social esteem and political importance.[42] This professional prestige was unquestionably connected to the abstract value attributed to science. Beyond that, however, it was the ideology of scientism and, more particularly, the expected social utility of German physicians that bestowed upon them both their much desired social role as custodians of the nation's health and their newly found esteem.[43]

The high self-image and lay perception of medical professionals as *Führer der Menschheit* (leaders of humanity) in the 1880s— the years during which Schallmayer completed his medical education and training—stemmed not only from the worldwide reputation of German laboratory medicine but also from the eminently practical advances in bacteriology associated with the name Robert Koch. The latter advances were especially significant in boosting the prestige and sense of social importance of medical men. Indeed it would be hard to overestimate the social impact of Koch's discovery of the tuberculosis and cholera bacilli (1882 and 1883) for the treatment and prevention of "two of the most pernicious enemies of mankind."[44] To be sure, the government as well as the public quickly recognized its value: almost immediately large sums of money were set aside for bacteriological laboratories and university chairs in the new field—no doubt a wise investment in the future health and productivity of the nation.[45] So much faith did some individuals have in the new

science that they seriously believed it possible to find a bac-
terium for every disease.[46] Medical progress appeared bound-
less, and physicians demigods. The euphoria over bacteriology
also swept the recently founded institutes of scientific (experimental) hygiene; indeed for more than a decade the province of
hygiene was virtually equated with the goals and aspirations of
the new science.[47]

The rise of bacteriology further reinforced the late nineteenth-
century German physician's self-image as custodian of the health
and well-being of society. This self-image was part of more than
a hundred year old tradition that lasted—with disastrous consequences—into the Nazi era.[48] But while all physicians shared
this tradition and benefited from the increase in prestige that
sprang from new medical discoveries, they had disparate intellectual backgrounds and chose disparate ways of fulfilling their
important social and political function of safeguarding and upgrading national health. Many believed that bacteriology and
related advances in serology and immunology afforded the best
means of combatting disease. Others, notably the renowned social hygienist Alfred Grotjahn (1869–1931), resented the usurpa-
tion of hygiene by the narrow field of bacteriology, and chose to
follow what, in the 1890s, was Virchow's nearly forgotten path of
examining the social factors contributing to ill health.[49] And finally, there were other medical professionals, among them
Schallmayer and many other eugenicists who, owing to their
exposure to fields of medicine that emphasized the role of heredity in the etiology of disease, argued that the surest way to
improve the general level of national health was to improve the
bodily constitution of all individuals in society.

While Koch's discoveries heralded a new dawn in the classification and treatment of infectious diseases, they held out relatively little promise for German neurologists and psychiatrists
seeking to explain neurological and mental disorders. Just prior
to and during the heyday of bacteriology (1885–1920), the new
university-based medical specialties of neurology and psychiatry
remained firmly under the intellectual tutelage of hereditarian-

ism. This tradition was not, of course, restricted to the two medical fields in question, but it was one which proved especially suited to "explaining" the allegedly functional diseases of the nervous system and brain. Although a strong commitment to and reliance upon hereditarian explanations of neurological and mental ailments is discernible as early as the 1860s,[50] by the 1880s one can speak of a veritable fetishism of heredity in German neurological and psychiatric circles. Physicians had at their disposal a large body of theoretical literature and a few clinical studies attesting to the fact that severe disorders such as mental illness, feeble-mindedness, criminality, epilepsy, hysteria, as well as less serious conditions such as nervousness and exhaustion, were often inherited.[51] Medical specialists usually chose to lump them together as manifestations of a weak or otherwise inferior hereditary constitution. By and large incapable of treating such ailments, Germany's nerve specialists and psychiatrists embraced instead two popular and related hereditarian theories to account for the wide variety of functional disorders: neurasthenia and degeneration.

The vogue of neurasthenia in both medical and literary circles on both sides of the Atlantic grew out of the writings of the American neurologist George M. Beard.[52] According to Beard, neurasthenia was a functional disease. Although it was purely somatic, neurasthenia—or nervousness—defied all attempts at anatomical localization. Weak nerves could lead both to insanity or epilepsy, but such developments could neither be predicted with scientific accuracy nor directly correlated.[53] In this assumption Beard and his fellow associates relied on the commonly accepted notion of the nervous diathesis as the physiological substrate of at least some nervous disorders.

Although Beard's findings on nervousness were available in Germany as early as 1871, the author failed to attract significant attention in Berlin, Zurich, or Vienna at that time. A decade elapsed before German-speaking neurologists and psychiatrists caught on; the 1881 German translation of Beard's *A Practical Treatise on Nervous Exhaustion (Neurasthenia)* more or less marked the beginning of the German reception of this form of hereditarianism. Once interested however, the German medical community honored Beard by publishing three separate editions of his text. The American neurologist could be proud that his theory was so favorably received in a country renowned for its science-based medicine.[54]

Among Beard's German-speaking apostles were the Leipzig neurologist Paul Julius Möbius (1853–1907); Rudolf Arndt (1836–1900), professor of psychiatry at the University of Greifswald; Otto Binswanger (1852–1929), professor of psychiatry at Jena; and perhaps the most distinguished of all, the expert on "sexual pathology" and psychiatry, Richard Freiherr von Krafft-Ebing (1840–1903). Despite differences in their professional concerns, all the above-mentioned men were especially preoccupied with the transmission of nervous disorders. As far as the inheritance of neurasthenia was concerned, they all focused on what Beard believed to be the single most important, if not the sole etiological factor in nervousness, the hereditary nervous disposition. *Erbliche Belastung* (hereditary taint)—a term frequently used by Schallmayer—became the catch-all phrase used by the German medical community to account for all pathologies of the nervous system.[55]

The German neurologists and psychiatrists even went beyond Beard in their emphasis on the nervous constitution. "Nowhere in medicine is the importance of heredity greater than in the case of nervous disorders," it was argued. "Compared to the role played by the hereditary constitution in the origin of nervous diseases, all other factors subside into the background."[56] For Möbius, at least one third of all mental illness was attributable to a hereditary nervous diathesis; simple nervousness was almost always inherited. Wilhelm Erb made the nervous disposition responsible for 75 to 80 percent of all reported cases of neurasthenia.[57] And Leopold Löwenfeld (1847–1924), a Munich specialist in nervous disorders (especially hysteria), conducted a survey of two hundred cases of neurasthenia which demonstrated that 75 percent of those troubled by nervousness and/or more serious related ailments inherited their pathological conditions.[58] The importance of the "soverign laws of heredity" as an explanation of nervousness could hardly be overestimated.

German medical experts viewed nervousness as the starting point for a wide variety of pathological conditions; similarly, the inherited neuropathic disposition was held responsible for the development of a whole series of serious nervous and mental disorders. According to Möbius the nervous constitution was pathological in and of itself. "Tainted individuals" could expect to suffer illnesses ranging from mild forms of nervousness to the most severe cases of idiocy:

> Anyone born into a tainted [erblich belasteten] family brings with him a tendency towards nervous and mental disease. This tendency manifests itself in certain peculiarities of bodily organization; its most common and simple expression is nervousness. In nervousness one can see the germ of serious pathological conditions. The latter evolves out of nervousness as soon as additional harmful stimuli induce such development.[59]

The psychiatrist Binswanger analyzed the role of the nervous system in a very similar light. Nervous disorders were part of "one large family"—erbliche Belastung could be used to account for all of them.

Neurasthenia as a particular form of hereditarianism would have been far less significant for Schallmayer and the future course of the German eugenics movement had it not been immediately linked to the then fashionable degeneration theory. First articulated by the French alienist Bénédict Augustin Morel (1809–1873) in 1857 and later adopted by German psychiatrists, the degeneration hypothesis virtually dominated the field of German psychiatry and related branches of medicine during the last quarter of the nineteenth and early years of the twentieth century.[60] The medical fascination with degeneration, along with neurasthenia to which it was intimately connected, was related to the lack of any therapeutic success in treating the mentally ill. The degeneration hypothesis provided an "explanation" for why the insane were so often incurable. Degenerates, it was argued, did not respond to treatment because they were part of an inherently diseased strain of the human race.

The degeneration theory undoubtedly also served a social and political function. The concept was essentially a classificatory system—a social classificatory system. *Degenerate* became the generic term for Imperial Germany's nonproductive or otherwise dangerous elements: the insane, the criminal, the feeble-minded, the homosexual, and the alcoholic. Such individuals, it will be recalled, were viewed as part of Germany's much-discussed soziale Frage. They detracted, at least psychologically, from the Bildungsbürger's idea of a well-ordered, harmonious, and conflict-free society. Considering the physicians' conservative worldview, their equation of degeneracy with social deviation from the bourgeois norm should not come as a surprise: by employing the socially stigmatic and scientifically pretentious word *degeneration*, German doctors possessed a useful means of classifying, separating, and ultimately controlling those who offended their social, political, and cultural sensibilities.

Morel's degeneration theory first began to attract the attention of the German medical community about a decade after the publication of his major treatise on the subject. It may be briefly summarized as follows: degeneration was the result of a deviation from a *type primitif* which existed before the biblical Fall. After the Fall, humankind was subjected to external influences such as climate, food, and customs the effects of which, together with God's punishment for Adam and Eve's disobedience, were inherited. This inheritance led to the formation of two distinct types of human species—the normal/healthy variety and the abnormal/sickly variety, that is, the degenerates.[61] Essentially nonhuman, degenerates allegedly possessed a combination of physical and mental traits which separated them from the healthy portion of the species. These abnormal traits were in turn transmitted from one generation to the next and with every generation became progressively worse. The result was the eventual extinction of the tainted families or groups.[62]

German degeneration theorists modified and updated Morel's work, carefully synthesizing it with prevailing theories of neurasthenia. According to Möbius, *Entartung* (degeneration) represented an "unfavorable hereditary deviation from type" which almost always entailed some change in the nervous system, usually in the brain.[63] Krafft-Ebing, perhaps the best known of the German degeneration theorists, drew an even more careful connection between neurasthenia and degeneration:

> Nervousness is only the mildest expression of an inferior organization of the central nervous system tending towards degeneration in the anthropological, biological, and clinical sense of the word. This can be deduced from the unbroken transition from . . . [nervousness to degeneration], from the side by side appearance of nervousness, and the most serious kind of neurotic degeneration, idiocy, in the same generation, and from the common cause of both pathological occurrences—hereditary taint.[64]

Having first rid Morel's degeneration theory of its religious inferences and language, Möbius and Krafft-Ebing helped popularize the concept in psychiatric circles through their influential pamphlets and treatises. By the end of the century, the term "psychic degeneration," a phrase frequently employed by Krafft-Ebing, had become part of German psychiatrist's standard medical vocabulary. Schallmayer most certainly heard the term used in university lectures and during his internship in a Munich psychiatric clinic.

Closely related to the problem of psychic degeneration was the "scientific debate" concerning the "born criminal." In Germany the heated discussion of this issue was touched off by the translation of the works of Cesare Lombroso, professor of legal medicine at the University of Turin. Lombroso, who beginning around 1890 gained a worldwide reputation through the publication of his notorious work *L'uomo delinquente* (1876), challenged the prevailing penal theory both in Italy and abroad with his *delinquente nato* (born criminal). According to the Italian professor, the born criminal represented an atavistic regression, a reversion to a more primitive stage of human evolution, whose criminal nature was easily recognizable by particular anatomical (pathological) traits. Because the criminal's deviant behavior was inborn—the result of an alleged hereditary disposition toward dangerous antisocial conduct—all attempts at rehabilitation by means of moral persuasion were doomed to fail. The best any penal system could do was to make sure that hereditary criminals, once apprehended, were never again allowed to pose a threat to society.[65]

No person did more to bring Lombroso's ideas to German psychiatrists, legal theorists, and judges than neurologist and psychiatrist Hans Kurella, German translator of Lombroso's most popular work. Reports and statistics indicating a substantial increase in criminal acts after 1870 convinced Kurella that Germany's penal code was simply impotent in combatting crime. The problem, according to the outspoken neurologist, was that German penal law emphasized punishment or reform of the criminal, neglecting the fact that such a strategy could have no possible effect on an individual destined by heredity to commit an asocial act. Kurella's 1893 treatise, *Die Naturgeschichte des Verbrechers*[66] (The Natural History of the Criminal) was designed to lay the foundations of a new science of criminal anthropology and criminal psychiatry, an undertaking that would truly create a "science" out of Germany's legal system.

Although many German psychiatrists and criminal specialists differed with Lombroso and Kurella about the degree to which one could recognize the born criminal by any specific anatomical characteristics, few doubted that such a person was more likely to deviate physically from the "normal type" than those not destined to steal or kill.[67] Even fewer questioned the accepted practice of lumping these tainted individuals together with the huge army of other types of mental degenerates. Indeed, the newer term *angeborene Verbrechernatur* (hereditary criminal nature) was just a synonym for the much older psychiatric concept of *moralischer Schwachsinn* (moral insanity), a form of mental degeneration.[68] Both terms were used to describe those "pathologically tainted individuals whose intelligence would suffice for the struggle for survival but who, because of their ethical inferiority, posed a danger both to themselves and society."[69]

While the term degeneration was most frequently employed by neurologists and psychiatrists in their attempt to explain various forms of antisocial behavior, the concept was gradually extended to include nonmental ailments as well. An individual might have a weak or otherwise "degenerate" constitution: a hereditary condition that would render him or her more susceptible to diseases like tuberculosis, for example. According to the clinical usage of the term *disposition* that by 1890 had been reformulated into a new full-fledged *Constitutionslehre* (constitution theory), the hereditary bodily constitution of all individuals varied in its ability to defend itself against both internal and external pathogenic agents, for example, bacteria. In the case of exposure to the tubercle bacillus, those individuals possessing a robust constitution would not become ill. Others, because of their overall weak or otherwise degenerate constitutions easily fell prey to these disease-producing irritants and became sick. The pathogenic agent was not the cause of the disease; it merely touched off its development. The true "cause" was the unfortunate victim with his or her deficient bodily makeup.[70] It was along similar lines that one practitioner defined the hereditary nature of tuberculosis as the "inheritance of certain bodily characteristics which provide the bacillus with the fertile soil needed for its continued growth."[71]

By the turn of the century there was hardly a known disease or an observable socially deviant action that was not included in the ever-growing list of *Degenerationszeichen* (signs of degeneration). The so-called hereditary tendency toward alcoholism and the disposition toward suicide were both seen as a sign of Entartung.[72] One German-speaking Hungarian physician, Moriz Kende, presented readers with an impressive catalog of diseases and phenomena that proved the reality of degeneration. It included the alleged increase in tuberculosis, scrofula, cerebrospinal meningitis, rachitis, anemia, diabetes, lung infections, heart diseases, cavities, the inability to nurse, short-sightedness, and the atrophy of the human breast observable in the general population of civilized (industrial) nations.[73] He also noted a rise in various forms of mental degeneracy. For Kende and other psychiatrists and neurologists, degeneration posed a serious and constant threat to the health of the community.

Degeneration and neurasthenia were perhaps the most fashionable and widely accepted forms of hereditarianism discussed in medical circles during the last quarter of the nineteenth century. As we have seen, they served important professional as well as political functions: both neurasthenia and degeneration theory enabled physicians to explain their obvious lack of success in curing mental disorders; degeneration allowed the practitioner to classify certain social parasites and social misfits as belonging to a pathological strain of the human race. This latter political function was particularly important for the subsequent development of German eugenic thought. Couched in the scientific/medical language of neurasthenia and degeneration, various types of asocial behavior came to be regarded by medical professionals as little more than bad hereditary traits. Because "degeneration" was seen as a straightforward medical problem rather than as a composite of social prejudices and fears, it seemed natural that many physicians committed to improving the welfare of the nation, offered purely medical rather than political solutions to the social question. Indeed, even some physicians not directly involved in the race hygiene movement called for marriage restrictions and sterilization of the degenerate. However, what separates Schallmayer from other physicians who advocated these and similar measures is his social Darwinist perspective and his denial that traits acquired during the life of an individual could be inherited. Schallmayer and other German eugenicists dislodged the degeneration theory from its Lamarckian origins and strictly medical usage, and placed it in a new social Darwinist context.

THE BIOLOGICAL COMPONENT:
THE POPULARITY OF SELECTION

Darwin's theory of evolution, especially as applied to human beings and human society, has always been recognized by historians as a key factor in the rise of the international eugenics movement. Indeed, the renowned English naturalist's theory of descent furnished the biological framework of eugenics and helped legitimize it as a political, social, and "scientific" movement—a point which eugenicists like Schallmayer never tired of emphasizing. Particularly important for understanding the intellectual origins of Schallmayer's eugenics is, however, the popularity that Darwin's theory of selection enjoyed in Germany during the four decades following· its introduction. The *Selektionsgedanke* (principle of selection) was publicized by two of Germany's most eminent biologists, Ernst Haeckel (1834–1919) and August Weismann (1834–1914), as well as by numerous self-styled Darwinian social theorists. Significant modifications of Darwin's theory by Weismann, and changes in the social meaning of Darwinian evolution during the 1880s and 1890s seemed to suggest to some that the "civilized" (white industrialized) nations of the world, and particularly the "fittest" classes of those nations (the educated middle classes), faced the danger of being overrun by the "uncivilized" and "unfit."

But what precisely was the link between Darwin's theory and the Selektionsgedanke? The answer is Darwin's mechanism of evolution, natural selection. It was this mechanism that separated the British naturalist's theory of the transmutation of species from all previous speculation on the subject.[74] His choice of the term *natural selection* to describe the means by which all species evolve is testimony to the great intellectual debt Darwin owed to English animal breeders and horticulturists. Their daily experience demonstrated that domestic breeds could be improved upon by selecting useful variations found among cultivated plants and animals and breeding them for successive generations. By employing the phrase "natural selection," Darwin wished to suggest that nature was capable of rendering change similar to but even more far-reaching than that of the breeder.[75] Indeed, in Darwin's view nature was constantly at work selecting those organisms of a species whose variations somehow enhanced their chances for survival and procreation relative to other members of the same species. In such a manner all living forms were said to have evolved one from another. Natural selection, Darwin assumed, ensured a kind of progress in the organic realm; remove it and all development would cease.

As is generally well known, Darwin did not attempt to deal with human or social evolution in *The Origin of Species*. It was not until twelve years later, in 1871, that his views on the role of natural selection for human and social development were made public in *The Descent of Man*. Darwin's own opinions on the subject were strongly influenced by the writings of the essayist W. R. Greg, Alfred R. Wallace, and above all by his cousin, the biometrician and eugenicist Francis Galton. During the 1860s these men published several articles in which they each asserted that civilization imposed a serious restraint upon the efficacy of natural selection for humankind. They did not reach the same conclusions from this alleged fact, however. On the whole Wallace remained optimistic about the future development of the species and its social institutions; Greg and Galton were extremely pessimistic. The latter two believed that modern society's humanitarian institutions were protecting the weak, the stupid, and the "unfit" at the expense of the strong, the talented, and the "fit." Unless some way could be found to effectively compensate for civilization's curtailment of natural selection, racial decay was inevitable.[76]

In the fifth chapter of *The Descent of Man*, under the section "Natural Selection as Affecting Civilized Nations," Darwin paid intellectual homage to his three fellow countrymen. John Greene has perceptively touched upon Darwin's ambivalent attitude regarding the notion of degeneration in civilized society.[77] Like Wallace, Darwin was convinced that our moral and intellectual nature set humans above other animals and was the positive result of natural selection. Like Galton, however, Darwin believed that humankind's moral nature impeded the continued efficacy of natural selection, and threatened to reverse all human progress.

Although Darwin was never fully able to reconcile this dilemma, he was consoled by his belief that the degenerative effects of modern culture did not go unchecked.[78] By and large, however, Darwin stressed Galton's line of reasoning more than Wallace's and took the theory of racial degeneration seriously:

> If the various checks specified in the last two paragraphs, and perhaps others as yet unknown, do not prevent the reckless, the vicious and the otherwise inferior members of society from increasing at a quicker rate than the better class of men, the nation will retrograde, as has too often occurred in the history of the world. We must remember that progress is no invariable rule. It is very difficult to say why one civilized nation rises, becomes more powerful, and spreads more widely, than another; or why the same nation progresses more quickly at one time than at another. We can only say that it depends on an increase in the actual number of the population, on the number of men endowed with high intellectual and moral faculties, as well as on their standard of excellence.[79]

Darwin suggested a eugenic solution to the problem of degeneration though much less vigorously than Galton:

> Man scans with scrupulous care the character and pedigree of his horses, cattle, and dogs before he matches them, but when it comes to his own marriage he rarely, or never takes any care. . . . Yet he might by selection do something not only for the bodily constitution and frame of his offspring, but for their intellectual and moral qualities. Both sexes ought to refrain from marriage if they are in any marked degree inferior in body or mind; but such hopes are utopian and will never be even partially realized until the laws of inheritance are thoroughly known. Everyone does a good service who aids towards this end. When the principles of breeding and inheritance are better understood, we shall not hear ignorant members of our legislature rejecting with scorn a plan for ascertaining whether or not sanguineous marriages are injurious to men.[80]

By lending his considerable scientific authority to the idea of selective breeding, Darwin did much to aid the cause of eugenics in Europe and the United States.

Darwin's views on the importance of natural selection for organic and social evolution, as well as his casual remarks about the desirability of human breeding, did not fall on deaf ears in Germany. In the two decades following the prompt translation of the *Origin* into German in 1860, numerous scientific books and articles were published that touched on the great English naturalist's evolutionary theory.[81] Although the overall reaction of the German biological community was mixed, many notable scientists such as Matthias Schleichen, Fritz Müller, Carl Gegenbauer, Ernst Haeckel, and August Weismann quickly became active supporters of evolution by means of natural selection.[82] But of all the above-named scientists, Weismann stands out as especially important in the history of German eugenics. Not only did his "modified" version of Darwin's theory give the selection principle an even greater role in organic and social evolution than did the author of *Origin* himself, but Weismann's views also provided the biological underpinning of the mature eugenic doctrine of Schallmayer and other German race hygienists.[83]

To be sure, Weismann did not begin his career with the intention of becoming champion of the "Neo-Darwinian" direction in biology. Trained both in medicine and zoology, the Freiburg embryologist eventually came to his position regarding the "all-sufficiency" of selection through his work on heredity. His developmental studies on insects, crustacea, and most importantly, his investigation of sex cells of the Hydromedusa during metagenesis made him extremely skeptical about the possibility of any organism being able to transmit characteristics acquired during its lifetime to the next generation. Darwin, it should be noted, found it necessary to incorporate an ever-increasing amount of so-called Lamarckian elements into the later editions of his *Origin*.[84] There were simply too many phenomena in organic nature which natural selection appeared unable to explain. In order to answer his many critics, Darwin introduced a wide variety of Lamarckian elements such as climate, food, and use and disuse of parts into the speciation process.[85] Weismann, although not the first to contest the inheritance of these Lamarckian factors, provided a viable theory and mechanism of heredity that appeared to render such factors not only superfluous but indeed impossible.

In his investigations Weismann noted that differentiation occurring in the production of all metazoa resulted in two types of cells, the reproductive and the somatic.[86] The big question remained: how could the first differentiation be explained? When a protozoan—a simple reproductive cell—divides, the result is two reproductive cells. How could a one-celled organism have given birth to a nonreproductive cell? For Weismann, the answer was found in the germ plasm. Variations in the original reproductive cell or groups of cells—that is, differences in their molecular or chemical structure—could upon division create not just the expected reproductive cells but nonreproductive ones as well. If this variation proved to be advantageous to the organism, it would be preserved by natural selection.[87] Assuming that part of the hereditary material of this varied reproductive cell remained unaltered, it could be passed down to future generations.

In short, what Weismann suggested in his first pamphlet on the subject, *On Heredity* (1883), and developed more fully in his later writings was the transmission of a hereditary substance through a "continuous and distinct tract" beginning with the very origin of life and proceeding from one generation to another. This "germ-tract," insofar as it occupied a "different sphere" from the somaplasm, was totally unaffected by what happens to the organism during its life.[88] Certain important revisions notwithstanding, this was the basis of Weismann's famous mechanism of heredity, "the continuity of the germ-plasm"—a theory wholeheartedly embraced by Schallmayer once it became known to him.

Weismann's theory emphatically excluded the possibility of an inheritance of acquired characteristics. If all changes in phylogenetic development occurred through alterations in the germ-plasm uninfluenced by any bodily changes in the organism, nei-ther the environment, the use or disuse of parts, nor indeed any other factor besides natural selection itself, could be of any sig-nificance for the evolutionary process. Moreover, Weismann maintained, there was no reason to accept an unproven hypoth-esis which was not even necessary for the theory of descent.[89] Even the existence of rudimentary organs, a perplexing phe-nomenon facing Darwin and one which he believed was only explicable in terms of disuse, could, according to the Freiburg embryologist, be satisfactorily explained without recourse to Lamarckian factors. In an attempt to explain the existence of rudimentary organs Weismann proposed his theory of *Panmixie*. The theory sought to account for the degeneration of an organ by means of the "suspension of the preserving influence of nat-ural selection."[90] He offered the following example of birds of prey:

> The sharp sight of these birds is maintained by means of the con-tinued operation of natural selection, by which the individuals with the weakest sight are being continually exterminated. But all this would be changed at once, if a bird of prey of a certain species was compelled to live in absolute darkness. The quality of the eyes would then be immaterial, for it could make no difference to the existence of the individual, or the maintenance of the species. The sharp sight might, perhaps, be transmitted through numerous generations; but when weaker eyes arose from time to time, these would also be transmitted, for even short-sighted or imperfect eyes would bring no disadvantage to their owner. Hence, by continual crossing between individuals with the most varied degrees of perfection in this re-spect, the average perfection would generally decline from the point attained before the species lived in the dark.[91]

In his magnum opus, *Vorträge über Deszendenztheorie*, Weismann went on to cite Panmixie, in conjunction with his principle of "Germinal Selection," as responsible for the short-sightedness and for the deterioration of the mammary glands in all classes of people, and for the weakness of muscles among members of the upper classes in modern civilization.[92] In his major treatise Schallmayer utilized both Weismann's example and his language to demonstrate both the possibility and the reality of racial degeneration.

In addition to the scientific reception of Darwin by eminent German biologists such as Weismann, the British naturalist's theory enjoyed an enthusiastic popular reception. As has been discussed at length in Alfred Kelly's extremely useful study, the rapid popularization of Darwin and Darwinism in Germany (indeed to the point where it became a sort of popular philosophy) was aided by, among other things, the country's strong popular science tradition.[93] As early as the 1870s such Darwinian terms as *Kampf ums Dasein* (struggle for survival) had "penetrated middle-class consciousness," and by the 1890s certain segments of the German working class had also become familiar with the basic tenets of Darwinism.[94] It is perhaps not an exaggeration to say that Darwin was more popular in the land of Goethe and Kant than in his native country.

One of the best known German popularizers of Darwin, and the most significant for Schallmayer's intellectual development, was the combative and controversial Jena marine biologist, Ernst Haeckel. In his address to the annual conference of the Association of German Scientists and Physicians in 1863 at Stettin, a speech viewed by Kelly as "the public debut of German Darwinism," Haeckel went far beyond the usually cautious Darwin in discussing the broader implications of the new theory.[95] Unlike Darwin, who, in his *Origin*, did not discuss human evolution for fear of criticism, Haeckel immediately included human beings as the end point of a long evolutionary chain connecting protozoan to people. Throughout his life—in his numerous popular texts and public lectures—Haeckel never tired of fleshing out the larger philosophical and social meaning of Darwinism. The Jena zoologist's rather dubious philosophical system, monism, was a direct outgrowth of his Darwinian outlook.[96]

For Haeckel, as his international bestseller *Näturliche Schöpfungsgeschichte* (The History of Creation) makes clear, Darwinism was synonymous with selection. It was, after all, Darwin's mechanism, natural selection, that revealed the "natural causes of organic development."[97] Prior to Darwin, perceptive biologists knew that some form of species transformation had taken place but they lacked any viable means of explaining it. Moreover, selection not only was responsible for evolution but also accounted for the alleged "Law of Progress,"[98] an idea Haeckel probably borrowed from Herbert Spencer.[99] Indeed Haeckel, like Spencer, *equated* evolution with progress; but whereas the latter viewed natural selection as just one of many factors responsible for progressive development, Haeckel singled out Darwin's principle as the most important, if not the sole engine of forward-directed organic and social change.

Yet Haeckel, like Darwin, also recognized that progress could be impeded, at least temporarily, by certain counterselective institutions in modern society which seemed to eliminate the "fit" and protect the "unfit." Modern military service and, by extension, contemporary warfare, were examples of such ominous institutions. For Haeckel,

> this and other forms of artificial selection practised in our civilized states sufficiently explain the sad fact that, in reality, weakness of the body and weakness of character are on the perpetual increase among civilized nations, and that, together with strong, healthy bodies, free and independent spirits are becoming more and more scarce.[100]

Another factor working against progressive development was medicine:

> The progress of modern medical science, although still little able really to cure diseases, yet possesses and practises more than it used to do the art of prolonging life during lingering, chronic diseases for many years. Such ravaging evils as consumption, scrofula, syphilis, and also many forms of mental disorders, are transmitted by sickly parents to some of their children, or even to the whole of their descendants. Now, the longer the diseased parents, with medical assistance, can drag on their sickly existence, the more numerous are the descendants who will inherit incurable evils, and the greater will

be the number of individuals, again, in the succeeding generation, thanks to that artificial *medical selection* who will be infected by their parents with lingering, hereditary disease.[101]

But despite the counterselective tendencies of medicine and the military—tendencies which Schallmayer later bemoaned even more forcefully—Haeckel remained optimistic; natural selection, "the strongest lever for progress and amelioration," he maintained, will triumph over all attempts by human society to limit its action.[102]

Insofar as Haeckel believed that struggle and selection were the major forces driving human history, he was not merely a popularizer of Darwin but was also a social Darwinist. Yet Haeckel's brand of liberal, optimistic social Darwinism was not Schallmayer's. Whereas the social Darwinism espoused by Haeckel, Spencer, and German social theorist Albert Schaeffle stressed the necessity of social progress and functioned more or less as a justification of the naturalness of a laissez-faire competitive society, a later variety did not. By the late 1880s and 1890s the necessitarian optimism that had been the hallmark of early social Darwinism began to dissipate, leaving a form that emphasized not the necessity but only the possibility of social progress. Instead of resting comfortably in the assurance that evolution would in the long run perfect humankind's physical, mental, and moral faculties, many late nineteenth- and early twentieth-century social Darwinists like Schallmayer denied the inevitability of such progress in the absence of some kind of conscious control over the reproductive capabilities of the "fit" and "unfit."[103]

There are, to be sure, several reasons for this growing pessimism regarding the inevitability of social progress and the growing demand that the state take an active role in regulating the nation's level of biological fitness, not the least of which was a general disillusionment in Germany with economic liberalism after the 1870s. Although the Great Depression period did not spell the end of economic growth, entrepreneurs did indeed find it more difficult to succeed during this time than they had in the past. Economic uncertainty unleased widespread social dissatisfaction and a growing tendency to embrace aggressively ideological political positions, particularly with regard to the proper social distribution of the allegedly dwindling national income. More generally, the economic slowdown resulted in an all-too-exaggerated malaise on the part of the German middle-classes. Bismarck's turn toward protectionism and his support of social legislation in the 1880s in part reflected this pessimistic psychological climate.[104]

This climate of social pessimism explains, at least partly, Weismann's appeal for social Darwinists after 1880. Along with Darwin, first-generation social Darwinists assumed that new characteristics acquired by an organism as a result of environmental change would be transmitted to future generations. This suggested, at least implicitly, that humankind's physical and mental traits could be improved by environmental changes. Weismann's theories, however, denied that such external influences could affect an individual's hereditary substance. The implication, for those predisposed to believe it for other reasons, was that the germ-plasm alone determined the fate of the individual and, by extension, that of the nation and race.[105] Since, as had been maintained by many, natural selection was no longer effectively able to weed out the bad or "unfit" germ-plasm (owing to the numerous cultural institutions hampering its operation), some form of human selection was necessary. As one German social Darwinist and race hygienist put it:

> It was Weismann's teaching regarding the separation of the germ-plasm from the soma, the hereditary stuff from the body of the individual, that first allowed us to recognize the importance of Darwin's principle of selection. Only then did we comprehend that it is impossible to improve our progeny's condition by means of physical and mental training. Apart from the direct manipulation of the nucleus, only selection can preserve and improve the race.[106]

Indeed for social Darwinists of the second generation—those who accepted Weismann's views on heredity and the "all-supremacy" of selection—eugenics was often seen as both a logical and necessary strategy to avert racial degeneration. In short, Weismann's theories provided the necessary biological justification for race hygiene.[107]

Late nineteenth- and early twentieth-century social Darwinism, the German medical tradition, and the Bildungsbürger's concern over the social question—these were the three most important influences responsible for Schallmayer's turn to eugenics. He attempted to grapple with the social problems resulting from Germany's rapid and thoroughgoing industrialization, he accepted the professional and intellectual norms fostered by the German medical community, and he embraced the "selectionist" variety of social Darwinism then fashionable among certain German biologists and self-styled social theorists. The impact of these contexts are immediately visible in Schallmayer's university education, medical training, early professional career, and first treatise.

II

THE RATIONALIZATION OF HEREDITY AND SELECTION: WILHELM SCHALLMAYER AND HIS FIRST EUGENIC TREATISE

THE EVOLUTION OF A EUGENICIST

Germany's first advocate of eugenics, Friedrich Wilhelm Schallmayer, was born on February 10, 1857 in Mindelheim, a small Swabian town in Bavaria about twenty miles southwest of Augsburg.[1] Although Wilhelm was one of eleven children, his father's prosperous carriage and wagon business made it possible for the talented and hardworking son to attend university.[2] Upon graduation in 1876 from the Humanistisches Gymnasium St. Stefan in Augsburg, Schallmayer, like many middle and upper-class youths, enlisted in the army as a one-year volunteer in order to fulfill his military obligations. After suffering a "loss of fitness for military duty," apparently owing to overexertion during a military exercise, any potential military career was over.[3] It is ironic that a man who later placed such emphasis on military fitness as a basis for separating hereditarily superior individuals from inferior stock was himself deemed "unfit."

Schallmayer's relatively brief and unhappy experience with the army most probably fostered his lifelong antimilitarism.[4]

While stationed in Würzburg, Schallmayer attended lectures at the Julius-Maximilians University. He dabbled in philology, German history, philosophy, and geography, apparently unable to settle on a definite course of study. Upon completion of his military duties and after two semesters at the University of Würzburg, Schallmayer, following the wishes of his parents, enrolled in the Faculty of Law at the University of Munich. Law, however, did not seem to hold his interest. Since Schallmayer's diaries, letters, and notebooks are either missing or destroyed, it is virtually impossible to offer an exact reconstruction of his intellectual development. One can only surmise that after a year of general studies at Würzburg, law struck him as being too narrow. Owing to his early interest in philosophy, which predated any formal course work in Würzburg, Schallmayer left Munich in 1879 and went to Leipzig to attend the lectures of philosopher and psychologist Wilhelm Wundt (1832–1920). He was now determined to make philosophy his life's work.[5]

Schallmayer's decision to study under Wundt is testimony to the former's reverence for the natural sciences and the scientific method. Wundt was hardly a typical German philosopher. Before coming to Leipzig in 1875, Wundt spent fourteen years at the University of Heidelberg working first in experimental physiology under Hermann von Helmholtz and later in "physiological psychology," a field he was instrumental in establishing. According to Wundt, philosophy, like psychology upon which it was based, was dependent upon the knowledge and methodology of the natural sciences.[6] This was far removed from the basic tenets of traditional German academic philosophy. Undoubtedly well acquainted with Wundt's prejudices and presuppositions, Schallmayer took courses in philosophy and anatomy during the three semesters he spent at Leipzig.[7]

Yet even the novelty of Wundt's revolutionary approach to the study of both psychology and philosophy did not totally satisfy Schallmayer. Although he was formally enrolled in philosophy, the future eugenicist soon turned his attention to the social sciences. In addition to the lectures he attended in the Faculty of Medicine (physiology and anatomy), the twenty-two-year-old Schallmayer began a systematic study of national economy, sociology, and socialism. He found the works of Albert Schaeffle, Herbert Spencer, and Karl Marx especially stimulating—a fact clearly observable in both his early and more mature writings.[8] Through his readings Schallmayer developed a healthy interest in the social question, undoubtedly the most critical issue facing anyone concerned with the social sciences. The question of how the proletariat could be peacefully integrated into society must have appeared all the more pressing because of the passage of the German Anti-Socialist Law in 1878, only one year before Schallmayer began his studies at Leipzig.

Evidence suggests that Schallmayer was receptive to socialism both while he was a student and for some time afterward. In the German context, however, such an attachment to socialism does not automatically imply a revolutionary or inherently progressive outlook. After laissez-faire liberalism was discredited by the depression of the 1870s, even segments of the German middle class (especially academics) began to ask themselves whether some variety of socialism might not be the best means of promoting the common good. This was, as we have seen, the view of many of Germany's university-based *Kathedersozialisten* (socialists of the chair) who were actively engaged in finding a viable solution to the social question.[9] Schallmayer never identified himself with "orthodox" socialism (Marxism) nor did he ever join the Social Democratic party.[10] The only brand of socialism acceptable to him was a form of state socialism as articulated by men such as Adolf Wagner and Albert Schaeffle. Schallmayer's "socialist leanings" do not betoken a radical or subversive political position vis-à-vis the state.

Perhaps realizing that he could never hope to earn a comfortable living by pursuing the social sciences, Schallmayer decided to turn to something more practical. In 1881, more than four years after he began his studies, Schallmayer enrolled in the

Faculty of Medicine in Munich. This time, however, he managed to complete a degree. Upon passing the state medical examination in 1883, Schallmayer became a licensed medical practitioner.

As was (and still is) common practice among German physicians fresh out of medical school, Schallmayer immediately set out to write a dissertation.[11] This he accomplished by securing an internship in the University of Munich psychiatric clinic then under the direction of Bernhard von Gudden (1824–1886), one of Germany's most eminent psychiatrists and personal physician to the mentally disturbed Bavarian King Ludwig II.[12] Von Gudden must have been greatly impressed by Schallmayer's clinical work in the university hospital's psychiatric ward, for he offered the young medical graduate the opportunity to become personal physician to Prince Otto von Wittelsbach, Ludwig II's brother, who was also insane. Schallmayer turned down this lucrative, prestigious position.[13] However, the offer alone stands as evidence against the suggestion that Schallmayer's views were in any way politically radical. Had he been considered politically subversive, he would certainly not have been offered such a sensitive post.[14]

We can merely speculate as to how Schallmayer's one-year internship at the psychiatric clinic might have influenced his later eugenic thought. He undoubtedly witnessed some of the most severe forms of mental disturbances classed under the heading "insanity," and had firsthand experience with many so-called mental defectives. Regarding the treatment and care of the insane and retarded, the young physician probably came away with the views of his teacher which, as one obituary of von Gudden reported, amounted to a "near complete resignation regarding the effectiveness of medical intervention."[15]

Although Schallmayer was already convinced at the time that psychiatry was not in the best interest of the human race, there is no evidence that Schallmayer entertained any eugenic solutions to the problem of mental degeneracy while working with von Gudden. In fact, after a lengthy discussion of the pros and cons of force-feeding the insane in his doctoral dissertation,

"The Rejection of Food and Other Disorders Regarding Food Intake by the Insane" (1885), Schallmayer reached the conclusion that such "mental defectives" must be kept alive.[16]

After completing his dissertation, Schallmayer spent the next year traveling to Berlin, Vienna, Greece, and Turkey before accepting a position as a physician on board a vessel headed for Brazil. It was at this time, in 1886, that he wrote the first draft of his first treatise. When he returned from Brazil in 1887 he worked as a general practitioner in Kaufbeuren, a small town forty miles from Augsburg, and soon after married the daughter of the city's mayor.

Because Schallmayer viewed his work as general practitioner as useless, if not indeed damaging to the improvement of the race, he decided to leave Kaufbeuren and specialize in urology and gynecology. At least in this area, Schallmayer thought, the prevention and treatment of disease would benefit not only the individual but also future generations. After a year of specialized training in Vienna, Leipzig, and Dresden, Schallmayer began a lucrative practice in Düsseldorf where he remained until 1897, except for the period 1894–96 when he again served as a ship's physician, this time on a German vessel bound for the Far East.[17]

GERMANY'S FIRST EUGENICS TRACT

Meanwhile in 1891, after a five-year search to find a publisher, Schallmayer was finally able to see his first book in print, *Über die drohende körperliche Entartung der Kulturmenschheit und die Verstaatlichung des ärztlichen Standes*. The slim forty-nine page treatise was republished under a slightly different title in 1895 and then again in 1898. Exactly why second and third editions were issued is not clear. Although Schallmayer reported (more than twenty years after the fact) that his book enjoyed numerous and lively reviews,[18] only six are known to me. Only one medical journal, the *Münchener medizinische Wochenschrift*, was among the six. Of the five others, all but one were affiliated with the Social Democratic party—a somewhat curious if not totally surprising state of affairs considering Schallmayer's proposal, advertised in the book's title, to "socialize the medical profession." These reviews notwithstanding, the treatise failed to make a significant and lasting impact during the 1890s. Despite the text's relative obscurity at the time it was published, it reveals the influence of the three contexts on his thought, and it offers several proposals that were later incorporated into his overall eugenic platform. But most important, the treatise shows for the first time the technocratic logic implicit in German eugenics: direct control over the differential birth rates of various national groups or classes in the interest of national efficiency.

In a manner reminiscent of Ernst Haeckel, Schallmayer began his work by comparing Darwin's theory to the Copernican revolution. Both were said to be "great achievements of the human spirit" that "destroyed an age-old *Weltanschauung*" while simultaneously providing humankind with a better understanding of itself.[19] For Schallmayer, however, this "Darwinian worldview" had less to do with the teachings of the English naturalist than with the fetishism of the selection principle as the instrument of human evolution and social progress—a view first popularized in Germany by Haeckel and Schaeffle.

According to this composite of views, evolution was an ongoing process; the bodily, intellectual, and social development of humankind was not yet complete.[20] Moreover, like Darwin and Galton, Schallmayer viewed all social progress as a function of bodily and mental improvement. To imagine that either our small-brained prehuman ancestors or present-day savages could create so complicated an edifice as modern industrial society seemed preposterous. To Schallmayer the high level of culture embodied in Western civilization was itself proof of just how far the human race (or at least part of it) had progressed during its long history. Yet progress, according to this view, was not inevitable. Whether the continuing process of organic and social development resulted in further perfection or improvement, or its opposite, degeneration, depended first and foremost on the efficient operation of natural selection.

The prognosis, as Schallmayer saw it, was not good. As noted previously, not only Darwin and Galton but also Haeckel expressed concern that modern civilization and its social institutions impeded the efficacy of natural selection. Convinced that "under the influence of our culture human selection deviates in many important respects from that which took place under natural or precultural conditions," Schallmayer posed what for him was the most critical question of all. Simply put, the issue involved was "whether the physical development of the human race, upon which the continuation of all cultural progress depends, is presently advancing or declining."[21]

Given Schallmayer's intellectual commitment to Darwinism and his practical experience in von Gudden's psychiatric clinic, his pessimistic assessment of the long-term value of therapeutic medicine is not surprising. Early in Part I of his treatise the future eugenicist accused his own profession of impeding the well-being of humanity:

> Of all our cultural achievements which impede natural selection with respect to the human race, medicine was the first to arouse my suspicion. This question was bound to trouble me since I was a medical student at the time. In fact, the joy I derived from my profession subsided as I became more and more convinced that, on the whole, the therapeutic application of medical science not only did not contribute to the perfection of the human species, but often even damaged it.[22]

Schallmayer legitimized his indictment of medicine by referring to the theory of natural selection, and the statistical and population thinking implicit in it. Medicine upset the ratio between the number of *begünstigtere Individuen* (more favored individuals) who succeed in reproducing, and the number of *mangelhaftere Organismen* (more deficient organisms) engaged in the same activity.[23]

For Schallmayer, differential birth rates among unequal organisms of the same species accounted for all evolutionary progress. "The shorter average life span of the weaker individuals," it was argued, "is the automatic steering control [necessary] for the continued transformation of each species, which, on the whole, leads in the direction of greater perfection."[24] Under natural conditions, the progeny of "favored individuals" in any given species necessarily constitutes a larger percentage of the total number of offspring than those with some kind of defect. Statistically speaking, weaker organisms are less likely to reach reproductive age than "robust" individuals. This, according to Schallmayer, was the process of natural selection. Modern medicine, however, tampers with the "natural" ratio existing between the "favored" and the "defective." Insofar as medicine extended the life span of "defectively constituted" or "generally weak" individuals, it enabled them to produce a greater number of offspring than they normally would under the "rule of nature." For Schallmayer, the resulting increase in number of defective individuals "did not lie in the interest of a favorable selection."[25]

Schallmayer's "defectively constituted" individuals were none other than the German degeneration theorists' *erblich Belasteten*—those people perceived to have some kind of socially dangerous or burdensome hereditary illness—individuals who, in one way or another, upset the harmony of the social body. Like Möbius and Krafft-Ebing, Schallmayer was concerned with the alleged increase in the number of people suffering from various forms of nervous disorders. He wholeheartedly embraced the idea, articulated by the German degeneration theorists, that the growing number of individuals troubled by nervous diseases was a consequence of the imbalance between the demands placed upon the nervous system by modern civilization and the nervous system's inability to effectively cope with the resulting stress. In Schallmayer's opinion, the average nervous system was merely too *leistungsunfähig* (inefficient) to keep up with the fast pace of industrial society.[26]

Simple nervousness, however, was not Schallmayer's main concern; the overriding problem remained the increased visibility of the insane. According to Schallmayer, modern psychiatry was itself in large measure responsible for this counterselective phenomenon. Forensic medicine assured that the insane need not serve the penalty for any crimes they commit since they could not be held legally responsible for their actions. In Germany's numerous asylums practicing psychiatrists protected such mental defectives from harming or even killing themselves. To make matters still worse, many of these deranged people were pronounced "cured" after a short period of time and then released from institutions. Once freed, nothing prevented them from returning to married life, or getting married and having children. Unfortunately for society, the offspring of these "cured" patients almost always inherited a "pathologically constituted nervous system" from either the paternal or maternal side. It was these *erblich belasteten* descendants who supplied the "best recruits for the army of the insane."[27]

Schallmayer did not neglect to draw the reader's attention to the consequences of such *scheinhuman* (superficially humane) care of the mentally defective for the efficiency of the German nation. "The insane," contended Schallmayer, "constitute an enormous burden for the state." Not only were they a financial drain on a country that had better things to do with its revenues but the care and maintenance of these nonproductive people also required the attention of a large number of persons who could be more productively employed elsewhere.[28] The worst thing, however, was the fact that all this expense did not succeed in reducing the number of these unfortunate victims, but rather enlarged it.

According to the German eugenicist, modern medicine also did the future of the race a disservice by prolonging the life of those afflicted with tuberculosis. Even Koch's vaccination designed to prevent people from contracting the illness was at best a mixed blessing. Since tuberculosis was a disease that primarily affected individuals with a "defective constitution," it had a selective effect; in the past, argued Schallmayer, it "cleansed humanity of a considerable portion of its weakest members."[29] Although humanitarian considerations compelled physicians to do everything in their power both to prevent and treat tuberculosis, the long-term consequences of more and more physically degenerate persons reproducing their own kind could not be taken lightly.

Couched in the terminology of efficiency, performance, and productivity, Schallmayer summarized his views on the so-called achievements of modern medicine by means of a comparison designed to appeal to his professional middle-class audience:

> Even if medical technology grew to such an extent that malfunctioning human organs could be safely replaced by healthy human, animal, or laboratory-produced ones, the following generations would not be more efficient, rather just the opposite: the more advanced therapeutic medicine becomes, the more succeeding generations will have need of it. Therapeutic medicine affects the improvement of national health in about the same way as poor-relief contributes to the improvement of national welfare. Both encourage an increase in the dependent [population]. . . . medicine, insofar as it aims at treatment rather than prevention, contributes nothing to the gradual advance of human productivity [*Leistungsfähigkeit*] and human happiness. *It aids the individual but at the expense of the human race.*[30]

His comparison of the counterselective effects of therapeutic medicine with that of aid to the poor reveals to what extent the medically degenerate and socially dependent were related in Schallmayer's mind. Both of these groups impeded the overall efficiency of the state; both represented a social and financial liability for the nation. Moreover, there was a large overlap between the two groups, as typified by the "pauper idiot"—individuals who, because of their mental deficiency, would forever remain part of Germany's *Lumpenproletariat*. Whether the behavior of such degenerates manifested itself as insanity, criminality, indigence, unemployability, or inebriety was of little importance. The defective portion of the population needed to be contained and controlled lest it undermine the fitness of the race and the Reich.[31]

Although Schallmayer was primarily intent on demonstrating the adverse relationship between modern medicine and racial efficiency, he did not neglect to point his finger at other "counterselective" institutions common to all modern nations. One such institution was the military. Assuming that the offspring of those selected for service were "on the average more valuable" to the nation than the progeny of individuals exempt from duty, Schallmayer maintained that the biological welfare of Germany was adversely affected by the reproductive advantage enjoyed by the *Militäruntauglichen* (militarily unfit). In the event of war, he argued, the most valuable portion of the male population is often killed or seriously wounded before it has a chance to leave its mark on the next generation. Those who remain at home have the opportunity to fill the job vacancies formerly occupied by men now on the front and hence are in a better situational and financial position to raise a large family. To make matters worse, even in peacetime the "unfit" father proportionately more descendants than do those required to defend the Reich, since the "fit" must give up their jobs to serve in the army. The net result of Germany's counterselective military institutions, as Schallmayer never ceased to reiterate, was the degeneration of the Volk.[32]

In addition to condemning both medicine and the military, Schallmayer also portrayed various contemporary social customs in a bad biological light. Most disturbing from his point of view was the custom of marriage dowries. Even when they displayed a high degree of physical and mental fitness, those women without a dowry corresponding to their social position were often forced to refrain from marriage and childbearing. This loss was further augmented by the fact that under the present system women with all kinds of hereditary deficiencies had no problem reproducing their own degenerate kind if their families were wealthy enough.[33]

Although inheritance was not mentioned by name in his first treatise, Schallmayer also followed Darwin and Galton in denouncing this time-honored institution in his later works. Inheritance, especially the commonly accepted practice of primogeniture, encouraged members of one of the fittest classes of society (the landed elite) to limit the size of their families in order to avoid parceling their wealth.[34] And in the all-too-frequent event that birthright did not coincide with a high level of hereditary excellence, the first-born son gained an unfair advantage over less-favored but more talented individuals in procuring the necessary material conditions for marriage and child-raising.

Of course Schallmayer's discussion of the counterselective effects of modern medicine was hardly original. By the time he wrote his treatise in 1886, Darwin, Galton, and Haeckel had already published their views on the subject. If we accept Schallmayer's word that he had neither read Galton nor the passage in Darwin's *Descent of Man* about the negative effects of modern civilization upon the efficacy of natural selection, we must either deduce that he had read Haeckel (whom he does not quote, although the text's language gives us strong reason to believe that he was familiar with Haeckel's works), or that these ideas, being "in the air," were simply synthesized by Schallmayer in a manner almost identical to those of his predecessors.

Fortunately, however, the one book which Schallmayer did cite in his first treatise provides us not only with the probable direct source of his views on the counterselective effects of medicine but also with a clear exposé of the logic underlying eugenic thought. This highly revealing source is a book entitled *L'hérédité: Étude psychologique sur ses phénomènes, ses lois, ses causes, ses conséquences* (1873) (Heredity: A Psychological Study of its Phenomena, Laws, Causes, and Consequences), written by the French psychologist and philosopher Théodule Armand Ribot (1839–1910).[35]

As is evident from the title of his treatise, Ribot set himself the task of coming to grips with the ubiquitous yet baffling phenomenon known as heredity. For the French psychologist, heredity was an irrefutable biological law which policed the animate world; it governed the external and internal structure, diseases, special traits, and acquired characteristics of all living organisms. In addition, the "blind fatality of heredity," it was argued, regulated both evolutionary progress and its opposite— degeneration. Incorporating elements of the then fashionable biological philosophies of history, Ribot made heredity accountable for the rise and fall of nations.[36]

What Schallmayer extracted from Ribot's lengthy text transcended the conventional medical wisdom regarding the heritability of "psychological abnormalities." He came away with a better understanding of just how significant heredity was in the life history of nations and races, and how human beings could administer the laws of heredity in order to control their own destinies. Indeed, Ribot aptly summarized the principle that would later become the cornerstone of all eugenic thought:

> . . . where man has discovered a law—that is, an invariable rule— which governs a group of phenomena, if these phenomena are within reach or come under his control, he can modify them, because he holds in his hands the mainspring that moves and governs them. Thus he is acquainted with the laws of heredity: he knows that they exist and act, notwithstanding many exceptions which mask their action. Can he turn them to account? Can he employ them for the perfection of his species? Let us put the question in clearer, more explicit terms. The starting point is a race of medium intelligence, morality and artistic and industrial capacity. The goal is a race, quick of comprehension and expert in action, well-disciplined, of gentle manners, and easily adapting itself to the complicated forms of civilization. . . . Can we, by means of selection and heredity, increase in a race the sum of its intelligence and morality?[37]

It is very revealing that Schallmayer later incorporated Ribot's emphasis on "selection and heredity" in the very title of his 1903 eugenic treatise, *Heredity and Selection in the Life-Process of Nations.* Heredity and selection, as two independent factors operating unhampered since the beginning of human evolution, brought the world's races, peoples, and nations to their present level of biological and social fitness. But this was a very time-consuming process. By rationally administrating the hereditary makeup of a population—by consciously selecting those individuals or groups seen to possess desirable "hereditary traits," and simultaneously selecting out those who embody undesirable, "degenerate" characteristics—it was possible to shape Germany's future as well as that of the world. What nature accomplished through the haphazard and drawn-out method of natural selection could be accomplished more efficiently and humanely by eugenics.

It is worth noting that in 1886, when Schallmayer wrote his first book, relatively little was known about "hereditary laws." Mendel's pioneering work in genetics, itself hardly a scientific basis for improving human stock, was not available until after 1900. At the time Schallmayer wrote his book he had not yet become acquainted with Weismann's hereditary theories. In fact, like most physicians before the turn of the century, Schallmayer was a Lamarckian—he believed characters and traits acquired during the lifetime of an individual could be transmitted to future generations. Although some biologists and physicians demanded a more critical approach to the study of heredity, what were generally understood to be the laws governing inheritance in the 1880s were little more than the belief that the sum total of a person's physical and intellectual traits—be they healthy or "diseased"—was passed on to the individual's descendants.[38]

Schallmayer bemoaned the fact that heredity, a subject of such medical and socal importance, had not yet become a true science.

> It is deplorable that so little of certainty is known regarding this very important and interesting question. One speaks about the laws of heredity. Certainly these do exist since all natural processes are subject to invariable laws. Accident occurs in the subjective, not in the objective world. The apparent irregularity of the hereditary process gives the impression that chance is operating. In reality there exists, even for these natural events, inviolable regularity. But these laws of heredity, which we must accept a priori as existing, are not yet known to us. We possess only hypotheses and guesses.[39]

Without a knowledge of the laws of heredity it was impossible to determine precisely whether a given disease was hereditary. More important, without a complete understanding of the hereditary process any appeal for a form of artificial or "rational" selection lacked sound scientific legitimacy. One could not easily institute laws prohibiting the marriage of "defectives" on the basis of "hypotheses and guesses."

Although Schallmayer recognized in 1891 that without a more scientific understanding of the laws governing inheritance his call for a rational selection of the German population would meet stiff opposition, he did not believe that this lack of knowledge was in itself a major impediment to improving hereditary fitness. Until such time that heredity becomes a science, health genealogies could provide enough information on the biological/medical history of German families to legitimate the creation of a new branch of hygiene dedicated to the betterment of the hereditary stock of the Reich.[40] Simply put, the goal of this new branch of hygiene was to impart a "rational influence upon human selection" in order to assure "the slow and steady increase in the number of robust individuals" and a decrease in the number of the "sick and weak."[41] Although not mentioned by name in the treatise, this new branch of hygiene to which he referred was none other than his later *Rassehygiene.*[42]

Schallmayer employed two main arguments to bolster his demand for a "rational" selection. First he appealed to medical considerations. According to Schallmayer some form of conscious selection was far more effective in eliminating disease than the thankless "Sisyphian labor" carried out by therapeutic medicine.

> It is infinitely easier to produce healthy and strong progeny from healthy individuals than it is to make a hereditarily tainted, diseased individual healthy and robust. Nature has at its disposal powers totally different than those of our "school learning." Even if science really advanced far enough to allow for the construction of "Homunculus in retort," humanity would still be better off to give first preference to nature. But why should we now, at a time when medicine can do nothing more than shabby patchwork, look down with foolish pride on the natural way towards improvement of the human body and mind?[43]

As we have seen, physicians believed they were faced with an increasing number of seemingly incurable mental and nervous diseases. For those members of the medical profession unwilling to throw up their hands in despair (at least in public), two courses of action (or inaction) were possible. One strategy employed by many of Germany's most prominent neurologists and psychiatrists was to label these orders "degenerative." Once an individual suffering from such an ailment was relegated into the category "degenerate," all medical responsibility ceased. No physician could "cure" a patient who was part of an inherently diseased strain of the human race. Another option open to doctors convinced of the heritability of almost all human traits was to embark upon a wholesale program of preventive medicine—to make sure so-called incurable diseases did not appear in the first place. This could be accomplished by means of a systematic control over "heredity and selection" within a given population, that is, by implementing a form of eugenics. As we shall see, the prominence of physicians in the membership and leadership of the German Society for Race Hygiene is testimony to the professional appeal that eugenics held for many members of the German medical establishment.

Schallmayer based his second argument for the adoption of a policy of "rational selection" on the inherent utility and cost-effectiveness of eugenics. He sought to demonstrate the efficacy of this new type of hygiene by subjecting both eugenics and education to a cost-benefit analysis. For Schallmayer, it was both more economical and more efficient for the state to control a child's nature than simply to rely on monitoring his or her educational milieu:

> The civilized state spares no sacrifice in its attempt to secure the fullest possible development of its descendants. The frailest youngster is burdened with compulsory school attendance. The state makes a large financial sacrifice towards this end and encourages parents to do the same; and rightly so. But attention to selection would be easier and would more profoundly affect the progeny. While schooling may indeed develop one's natural faculties ... it can in no way compensate for defective mental or physical traits. ... The perfection of mental and physical characteristics which, owing to cultural progress has become absolutely essential, can in no better fashion be procured for future generations than through the *application of human reason to human selection.*[44]

Although the German educational system served to instill the virtues necessary to bolster existing political and social relations,[45] it might be more reasonable simply to breed politically and socially desirable traits. A policy of rational selection could go a long way towards eliminating the reputed ever-increasing number of "moral degenerates" hereditarily immune to the ethical imperatives preached in the German classroom.

From his discussion in Part I of both the imminent threat of degeneration and the counterselective institutions of modern civilization, Schallmayer then turned in Part II to an elaboration of a few proposals designed to set Germany back on the road to biological and social progress. For Schallmayer, biological decline was not, as some social theorists professed, humanity's *unabwendares Schicksal* (inevitable fate). Modern society could alter or offset many or all counterselective practices with "sacrifices that are small compared to those the modern state undertakes for less noble ends."[46] In fact, the prevention of degeneration was not merely desirable; it was an ethical imperative. The state, Schallmayer contended, had a moral duty to protect its biological vitality. In the long run the hereditary fitness of a nation's population was its most important inheritance. Yet the state did not exploit its valuable bequest wisely; instead, as Schallmayer remarked (employing a metaphor designed to point out the inherent similarities between people and property as economic resources), it wastefully depleted its "entail."[47] Only by acting promptly could the modern state put a halt to the needless squandering of its biological inheritance and thereby avert economic, social, and political downfall.

Schallmayer suggested a definite course of action. The first step in a strategy of rational selection entailed making the question of heredity "the object of extensive observation."[48] By this Schallmayer meant the compilation of an exhaustive and reliable set of national statistics on certain select diseases and pathological conditions. The young author believed this information would supply the raw data necessary for a scientific study of heredity. In addition, the process of collecting medical statistics would, he contended, necessarily lead to the formation of genealogies by which the eugenic advisability of a marriage could be ascertained.

The responsibility for recording and codifying the nation's stock of pathological traits fell to Schallmayer's professional colleagues, the physicians. According to Schallmayer's plan, all individuals, regardless of their present state of health, would be issued an official two-sided *Krankenpaßkarte* (health passport) by the state. Side one was to contain an exact description of the holder, considerably more detailed than an ordinary travel passport. Schallmayer expected that this information would serve not merely to identify the individual but also as indispensable data for statistics on the inheritance of "nonpathological" traits.[49] On the reverse side ample room would be provided for an individual's personal physician to enter any and all cases of a disease suffered by the passholder for which the state amassed statistics. The physician also had the duty to record on side two, cases of any illness which he believed might lead to the confirmation of a significant hereditary trait.

Under this proposal individuals with entries on their card would be compelled to turn in their passports once a year to their personal physician. He, in turn, had the obligation of delivering the passports to a local health office to be stored and processed.[50] After that, as Schallmayer saw it, a proposed central health ministry was to finalize the business of taking inventory of all serious hereditary disorders in the Reich by compiling the data collected from all the local offices into a comprehensive set of medical statistics. These statistics, once compiled, would then be analyzed and evaluated. The entire process of rationalizing German health records would be directed and supervised by Germany's medical practitioners.

While Schallmayer's plan was a necessary prerequisite for a policy of "rational selection," it alone was not the sum total of his conception of heredity as the "object of extensive observation." Implicit in this statement was a novel understanding of heredity as something to be known by all people. Heredity, once a subject discussed only by specialists, was no longer to be confined to the limited space of academic discourse; Schallmayer wanted it to enter the public domain and become, so to speak, a national preoccupation. Before action could be taken to stop the process of biological decline, words such as heredity, heritability, trait, etc., had to become part of the layperson's active vocabulary. From the eugenicist's point of view it was imperative that individuals become acutely aware of the difference between people, that is, "biological differences." Strong lines of demarcation between the strong and the weak, the talented and the stupid, the moral and the immoral, the "healthy" and the "pathological" had to be made by all Germans. But most important, people needed to recognize that an immutable "law," not susceptible to alteration but certainly subject to human control, governed the appearance and reappearance of these differences. In short, Schallmayer demanded that all Germans "know" heredity and take it "into account."

At no time was it more important for an individual to take heredity "into account" than when choosing a future spouse. Earlier in his work Schallmayer had lamented that nonbiological considerations such as money often determined not only if and when people married but also whom they married. From the standpoint of the biological vitality of Germany, this was a pernicious state of affairs. Schallmayer hoped that once the individual health passports developed into a form of medical genealogy, the latter would be used by prospective couples and their parents, "when they stood before the question of whether or not they should become part of the family."[51] Schallmayer fully expected such genealogies to provide the basis for a rational sexual selection that would not only improve the couple's chance of having mentally and physically sound offspring, but would simultaneously upgrade the hereditary fitness of the nation.

The health passport would serve yet another purpose in addition to its functions of providing the raw data for a science of heredity and the necessary biological/medical information needed to rationally select a suitable marriage partner. On the basis of the medical testimony on the passport, the state could, in the interest of the individuals involved as well as its own, prevent people from marrying. According to Schallmayer, a certificate of health should accompany all marriage petitions; if, for some reason, one or both of the parties were afflicted with a disease that would affect or be transmitted to future generations, the state had the right to intervene to prevent such a perilous union.[52]

In many cases the denial of permission to marry would merely be temporary; in some instances, however, *raison d'état* would demand it be permanent. A man infected with syphilis or gonorrhea, for example, need not, indeed should not remain celibate his entire life. He had only to wait until a physician pronounced him "cured." Once cured of the infection, the individual was free to marry—provided of course that there were no other medical objections to the union. But there were some hereditary disorders for which there were either no known remedies or which, even if treatable, were said to impart irreparable damage to the individual's germ-cells. According to Schallmayer, carriers of such diseases or *Krankheitsanlagen* (diseased traits) should forever be barred from the bond of matrimony.

Unfortunately, Schallmayer chose not to specify precisely which afflictions warranted such drastic state intervention; he simply made the vague recommendation that those people should be prevented from marrying whose "diseases and diseased traits, based on the sound results of future study proved to be hereditary and especially damaging to future generations."[53] Despite his reluctance to be specific about just which disorders were grounds for lifelong celibacy, there can be little doubt that Schallmayer expected his proposed set of statistics to demonstrate the heritability of a wide variety of mental and physical disorders. Any other interpretation does not render plausible his assertion that if the state refused one to two percent of all sexually mature Germans the right to reproduce (by denying them permission to marry), only the most injurious traits could be eliminated in the first generation. If, however, as Schallmayer suggested, the government continued to force the same percentage of all "unfit" individuals of marriageable age to remain single, most if not all defective traits would eventually disappear. Such a happy state of affairs was inevitable, since with each succeeding generation, fewer diseases and disorders would be present in the population.[54]

Schallmayer did not delude himself into thinking that his "hygienic" strategy for improving Germany's biological efficiency would be readily accepted by large segments of the population or speedily put into practice by the state. Although the text is not clear, Schallmayer probably expected that the interest generated by the heredity question would lead to a general recognition of the need for laws barring the defective from marriage, especially after statistics on the transmission of a wide variety of diseases became readily available. Schallmayer clearly perceived that a heavy does of *Belehrung* (instruction) was a necessary prerequisite for any state intervention. The public, it stood to reason, had first to become accustomed to "taking heredity into account." Yet despite the realization that the time for a full-scale policy of rational selection was not yet at hand, Schallmayer remained optimistic; he believed that the institutionalization of eugenically motivated marriage restrictions need not always remain in conflict with the ethical sensibilities of the German people.[55] Given the proper education and encouragement, individuals could be expected to embrace a new moral code, which Schallmayer later termed "generative ethics."[56]

Health passports, medical genealogies, marriage restrictions— these were the "direct" hygienic means by which Schallmayer sought to monitor human selection. He did, however, touch briefly upon another proposal designed to offset the counterselective tendency of Germany's military institutions. Individuals who were exempted from military service owing to some mental or physical defect, but who were still capable of earning a reasonable income, should become subject to a twenty-year *Wehrsteuer* (military tax). The expressed purpose of this military tax was to assure that men deemed unfit for military service (the assumption being that those exempt were, more often than not, "biologically inferior") would not continue to enjoy an economic, and hence reproductive advantage over the "fitter" in arms. The tax would make it more difficult to raise large families or ever marry. But as was the case with his "hygienic" proposals, Schallmayer did not lay out all the specifics of the particular plan. He neglected to mention, for example, just what percentage of the individual's earnings should be taxed, stating only that he favored a progressive tax based on income with exemptions for the poorest of those rejected from military service.[57] Nor did he state whether the tax should vary according to the particular kind of defect possessed by the individual. For Schallmayer the important point was that some sort of control over the birthrate of this particular "unfit" portion of the population be exercised. Experts would undoubtedly hammer out the details at some future date—and these experts would probably be physicians.

After delegating such a critical and sensitive role to medical practitioners in his eugenic scheme, Schallmayer felt compelled to evaluate realistically the suitability of physicians for the job. Were German doctors presently in the professional and social position necessary to effectively and efficiently lay the groundwork for a policy of rational selection? In chapter 1 we examined the intellectual tradition and social background of Germany's medical establishment. Whereas the emphasis placed on hereditarian explanations of disease in academic medicine and the strong German tradition of "political medicine" would have probably assured a favorable intellectual reception for his proposals among German physicians, Schallmayer asserted that their precarious economic situation virtually precluded them from becoming the true guardians of the nation's health and well-being. The physicians' task of rationalizing and codifying the nation's stock of hereditary traits demanded that they enjoy a measure of financial and social independence not compatible with the laws of the free market.[58]

> The proposed organization of statistics cannot, in my perhaps erroneous opinion, properly be executed under the present-day private medical system. It requires, as I see it, the transformation of the entire medical profession into a class of civil servants.

Only when the physician is no longer a businessman and is exclusively a civil servant will he both want and be able to undertake the duties which the proposed organization of statistics demands of him. Temporarily, as long as the information leading to the study of heredity serves pure scientific ends, private physicians can be charged with the task, although it would certainly never be possible to win over all of them to this idea, and the survey would not attain the degree of accuracy that it would under a state organ, since only the latter is both largely independent of the public and subject to control.

Later, however, when the information collected by the physician not only serves scientific, but, under circumstances, is also used to make practical decisions regarding the fitness of certain individuals for marriage, private physicians can no more be entrusted with these decisions than they can with those concerning military fitness or unfitness.[59]

It is easy to see why Schallmayer believed that transforming private physicians into medical civil servants would improve their effectiveness in a program of rational selection. Unless employed by the state as either a university professor, county health official, or military physician, medical doctors were virtually totally dependent on attracting and retaining patients for their livelihood. What doctor could hope to hold on to a patient after labeling him or her "unfit" for marriage? What young roué would continue to seek the advice and professional help of his personal physician knowing that the latter was under obligation to publicly expose his sexual exploits? And, finally, how many private medical practitioners were so self-sacrificing that they would concentrate their efforts on preventive medicine when treatment was their only source of income? Clearly, physicians were under financial pressure to cure and cover up disease; only after medical practitioners gained a sufficient measure of independence would they have the "power and interest" to prevent diseases from occurring.

Although Schallmayer formulated his plan to nationalize the medical profession with the specific intention of laying the groundwork for the complete rationalization of heredity and selection, his proposal also reveals the degree to which the author was aware of and concerned about a number of significant developments affecting the German Ärztestand (medical profession). The subjection of the medical profession to the laws governing the free market, coupled with both an increased number of physicians relative to the entire population, and the growing dependency of physicians on the good will of the newly established health insurance companies, threatened to seriously endanger the financial security and social status of German medical doctors. Given both the high degree of material security and the enviable social position enjoyed by Germany's Beamtenstand (civil servants),[60] Schallmayer's suggestion that physicians become civil servants was designed, whether consciously or unconsciously, to further enhance the power and prestige of the medical profession.[61]

Although, as Schallmayer fully realized, most physicians were still unfavorably disposed towards the idea of giving up their private practices and becoming subject to bureaucratic control, however noble the cause, at least a few members of the medical community were receptive to some limited form of increased government regulation of the medical profession.[62] All physicians, not just university-based medical researchers, the argument ran, must be made to serve the common (national) good, since health was not merely a private but an inherently political matter. As one medical doctor expressed it, "in the never-ending drive between rival nations for predominance, an increasing measure of government control or activity in the area of health will serve as a weapon in the struggle for survival to preserve and strengthen national power."[63]

Schallmayer's own views on the political significance of health can best be seen in an 1899 article entitled "A Ministry of Medicine." Exasperated by the absence of a national Ministry of Health in Germany[64] with powers and responsibilities equal to the other Reich ministries, he sought to convince those in authority of the national importance of establishing such a body, directed and staffed of course by physicians:

Who would have the nerve to maintain that a minister exclusively responsible for the health and strength of the bodily organism for all citizens administers goods [*verwaltet Güter*] less valuable than those of an agricultural, trade or railroad minister? The state has above all an economic, but also an ethical, and to a certain degree a military interest in improving the physical and mental efficiency of its citizens as well as alleviating their pain and prolonging their life. First of all, it is the task of government to see to it that disease and accidents as well as all other influences that weaken physical and mental productivity are prevented; and second of all, that the injuries are healed as quickly and as fully and with the least amount of pain as possible. For the same reasons the state should take up the task of insuring that seriously diseased traits or otherwise disadvantageous bodily constitutions are not passed on to future generations.[65]

Again, the emphasis here is on population as a natural resource which becomes even more valuable when in "good health." This quotation lays bare the relationship between medicine, health, and national productivity in Schallmayer's thinking. Rational selection was merely the form of medicine that could most efficiently and effectively boost national productivity. And physicans, being health experts, were the most likely candidates for the task of monitoring the Reich's level of biological vitality upon which national strength and power was based.

Schallmayer's plea for a nationalization of the medical profession in the interest of both physicians and the Reich went unheeded. Germany never undertook the compilation of the type of medical statistics envisioned by him; nor did the state pay any attention to Schallmayer's proposal for eugenically grounded marriage restrictions. In fact, as was previously mentioned, Schallmayer's short treatise had little impact. Only after the publication of Schallmayer's *Vererbung und Auslese* in 1903 was Germany's first eugenic tract rescued from oblivion.

Yet the book gives the critical reader a window through which to observe the intellectual and social genesis of eugenics. We have seen how, couched in the biomedical terminology of degeneration, Schallmayer saw the increased visibility of certain social types as socially threatening, fiscally damaging, and potentially politically dangerous. The newly acquired Darwinian perspective and language afforded Schallmayer novel analytical tools to tackle the social question by transforming it into a biomedical one. And the social and intellectual tradition of Germany's medical profession, to which of course Schallmayer belonged, made it possible for the author to view national wealth as a function of national health. As Schallmayer's text brings to light, what later became known as eugenics was in fact a locus at which three separate contexts intersected in time and space to form a new discipline and discourse.

But perhaps more important, the author's work reveals the administrative, managerial logic at the very foundation of eugenics. Behind Schallmayer's intention to apply "human reason to human selection" was a technocratic conception of population as a natural resource which, in the interest of national efficiency, should become subject to some form of rational control. We have also seen the degree to which the economic language of efficiency and productivity permeated Schallmayer's eugenic discourse, a language which had its roots in German cameralist and statist traditions as well as industrial capitalism. It is indeed revealing that the utopian vision depicted in Edward Bellamy's *Looking Backward* so captured the attention and approval of Schallmayer.[66] Bellamy's future socialist society placed a premium on productivity, efficiency, and proper management of human resources—in short, it was a meritocracy. As Schallmayer put it, such a society is a place where "the effectiveness of natural selection is not curtailed."[67] Through a policy of rational selection Schallmayer sought to create the kind of meritocratic state envisioned by Bellamy. And one further coincidence: the hero of Bellamy's novel who describes the virtues of the new order is a physician!

III

THE KRUPP COMPETITION OF 1900 AND SCHALLMAYER'S AWARD-WINNING TREATISE

With the exception of one short article not directly pertaining to eugenics, the ten years following the composition and subsequent publication of Schallmayer's *Über die drohende körperliche Entartung der Kulturmenschheit* did not witness any further treatment of the problem of degeneration by the author.[1] Because of the time spent acquiring the necessary background to specialize in urology and gynecology, and the long hours devoted to his medical practice in Düsseldorf, Schallmayer at first had little opportunity to give further written expression to his fears of biological decline. Only in 1897 had the forty-year old Schallmayer acquired sufficient means to settle down in Munich as a *Privatgelehrter* (independent scholar) and devote his full attention to spreading the eugenic gospel in Germany.[2] But even then he did not immediately demonstrate much scholarly initiative, perhaps owing to his disappointment over the absence of widespread public acclaim for his eugenic proposals. The time was not yet ripe, Schallmayer probably thought, for a "scientific" solution to Germany's social and political problems—or so it seemed until an unprecedented event in 1900 gave him good reason to think otherwise. The Krupp competition of that year marked a turning

point both in Schallmayer's personal career and in the attention
paid to eugenics in Germany.

THE ORIGINS AND ANNOUNCEMENT
OF THE COMPETITION

At first glance it may seem to be merely an accident of history
that the famous/infamous House of Krupp should have unwittingly been the midwife in the birth of a new, allegedly "scientifically based" eugenics movement. An examination of the history of the competition, however, reveals that the owner of
Europe's leading cast-steel and armaments firm might well have
had personal and political reasons for wishing to sponsor the
contest which Schallmayer later won.

Friedrich Alfred Krupp (1854–1902), the initiator and sponsor
of the contest,[3] was the grandson of the founder of the industrial
dynasty.[4] Although the Essen-based family prospered as mer-
chants and tradesmen from the time the very first Krupp, a
refugee, arrived at the city gate in 1587, the modern *Firma
Friedrich Krupp* was established just after the Napoleonic Wars.
At this time Friedrich Alfred's grandfather, Friedrich Krupp
(1787–1826), decided to cast his lot with the forces of industrial
modernity and invest his family's fortune in the production of
cast steel, a metal hitherto manufactured only in England.[5] In
the long run, however, it was the foresight, ruthlessness, and
good timing of the sponsor's father, Alfred (1812–1887), *der
grosse Krupp* that transformed the modest House of Krupp into
an economic force with which the newly created German Reich,
and ultimately the world, had to reckon.

The secret behind Alfred Krupp's economic fortune was his
decision to utilize the firm's first-rate cast steel in the production
of weapons of war. Traditionally, weapons such as cannons and
guns were made of bronze, and it took Krupp years of prodding
to convince the hardheaded, conventional generals of Prussia's
War Ministry of the military desirability of steel. Ultimately,

however, several years after the recognition bestowed upon Krupp at the 1851 London World's Fair for his steel barrel field gun, Prussia did take notice of the man who would later become Germany's favorite son.[6] When his cast-steel munitions proved their superiority on the battlefields of Sedan as well as on the streets of Paris, the personal success of Alfred Krupp and his now moderately large industrial concern became forever tied to the fortunes of the newly founded German Reich.[7]

During the 1860s and 1870s Krupp acquired a near monopoly over the requisite materials and machines for his tools of war. This monopoly does not, however, in itself account for the firm's remarkable degree of productivity and power. Krupp's near-total control over his *Kruppianer*, as his workers were called, was at least as important to the Krupp dynasty. In fact, the political subservience and economic efficiency achieved by Krupp's paternalism so impressed Bismarck that the latter modeled his own social welfare legislation on Krupp's conservative revolution in worker control.[8] Concerned only to perpetuate the industrial dynasty's fortune "for times perennial," Krupp established what was essentially a company town in the middle of Essen. In return for their absolute loyalty to the firm, Krupp workers were provided with housing as well as health and old-age insurance—a measure rooted in the idea that only when a worker's minimal requirements were met would he be in the physical and mental condition to produce at full capacity. Krupp thus managed to gain control over "his men," thereby preventing the development of any incipient working-class consciousness or political activity on the part of his labor force. His fear and hatred of both the Social Democratic party and the trade unions were legendary. To make sure that his more that 50,000 workers did not become indoctrinated with dangerous ideas, Krupp even had their trash cans checked for socialist newspapers and literature.[9]

When Alfred Krupp died in 1887, Friedrich Alfred was only too anxious to continue his father's role as master and protector of the firm. Like his father, the well-being of the firm was closest to Fritz's heart. But unlike his father, he did cultivate one outside interest: zoology. The new master of the House of Krupp even fancied himself as a marine biologist.[10] Prevented by his father from actively pursuing his interest in biology while still an adolescent, as a grown man he indulged himself in the study of aquatic life and oceanography, apparently with some limited measure of professional success.[11] Whether or not, as one Krupp biographer suggests, Fritz actually received an invitation by the marine biologist and founder of the famous Zoological Research Station in Naples, Anton Dohrn (1840–1909), to participate in the researches undertaken there, he undoubtedly remained in contact with Dohrn and his associates over the years.[12] Krupp was so convinced of the importance of the scientific work undertaken at Naples that he contributed 100,000 marks toward the construction of a biological laboratory at the site.[13]

Given his interest in deep-sea life, Krupp wanted to involve Germany's most distinguished marine biologist and one of its most controversial public figures, Ernst Haeckel, in his plans for the contest. The subsequent history of the German eugenics movement owes much to this decision. By 1890 Haeckel had long since become interested in problems which transcended his careful investigations of the medusa. It was Haeckel's role as apostle of Darwin in Germany that accounted for his extraordinary popularity and notoriety among his numerous admirers and enemies. And just as the original Christian apostles did not merely preach the message of Christ, but also interpreted it to fit the needs of the early church, so too did Haeckel go beyond a mere explication of Darwin's theory of descent and sought to interpret its social and political meaning.

Part of the social and political meaning that Haeckel attributed to Darwinism was its incompatibility with socialism— an interpretation which undoubtedly appealed to Krupp. Beginning in 1877, in his famous debate with the eminent German pathologist Rudolf Virchow at the Fiftieth Conference of the German Association of Naturalists and Physicians,[14] Haeckel sought to publicly sever the link between Darwinism and Social Democracy that had been forged by several prominent German socialists. During the 1860s and 1870s Social Democratic leaders such as Friedrich Albert Lange, August Bebel, and Karl Kautsky—to name only the most important—embraced Darwinism and viewed it both as a legitimation of the inevitability and desirability of socialism, and as a justification for materialism and atheism.[15] Haeckel, however, considered socialism to have "the most dangerous and objectionable character which, at the present time, any political theory can have," and asserted during the 1877 debate that Darwinism

is anything rather than socialist! If this English hypothesis is to be compared to any political tendency—as is, no doubt possible—that tendency can only be aristocratic, certainly not democratic, and least of all socialist. The theory of selection teaches that in human life, as in animal and plant life everywhere, and at all times, only a small chosen minority can exist and flourish, while the enormous majority strive and perish miserably and more or less prematurely. . . . The cruel and merciless struggle for existence which rages throughout all living nature, and in the course of nature *must* rage, this unceasing and inexorable competition of all living creatures, is an incontestable fact; only the picked minority of the qualified "fittest" is in a position to resist it successfully, while the great majority of the competitors must necessarily perish miserably. We may profoundly lament this tragical state of things, but we can neither controvert it nor alter it. "Many are called but few are chosen." The selection, the picking out of these "chosen ones" is inevitably connected with the arrest and destruction of the remaining majority.[16]

Haeckel's uncompromising antisocialist interpretation, while certainly reflecting his own personal political position, was also designed to promote the teaching of Darwin's theory of evolution in the public schools by demonstrating that it presented no threat to the political status quo.

Given these views Krupp was undoubtedly delighted when the biologist Heinrich Ernst Ziegler (1858–1925) informed him of Haeckel's willingness to preside over a written contest designed to demonstrate, once and for all, that the new biology was anything but *staatsfeindlich* (a threat to the state).[17] Sometime before January, 1900 (the exact date is not known) the details of what became known as the Krupp *Preisausschreiben* were ironed out.

"Toward the advancement of science and in the interest of the Fatherland," Krupp donated 30,000 marks to be used in a contest to answer the question: "What can we learn from the theory of evolution about internal political development and state legislation?"[18] Wishing to remain anonymous, Krupp did not involve himself personally with the administration and execution of the contest; it appears that Ziegler, who was asked to be a judge for the contest, did much of the work. Krupp did, however, choose to formulate, in collaboration with his "scientific friends," not only the general question but also a number of specific guidelines pertaining to both the form and content of the entries.

It was not sufficient for those interested in the exceedingly generous 10,000 marks first prize simply to discuss the political and social meaning of Darwin's theory. In addition to answering the general question, all participants had to take a stand on a number of issues. First, every contestant was expected to discuss the importance of heredity in the evolutionary process and to take sides on this hotly debated issue. In effect, the rules required a contestant to choose between Lamarckism or Weismannism. Since the political lesson that could be drawn from evolutionary theory varied greatly depending upon whether or not one believed in the inheritance of acquired characters or traits, it was essential to clearly articulate and defend a position on the subject. Moreover, those participating in the contest were asked to comment on the relative importance of nonhereditary factors such as customs, tradition, and education in the process of social evolution, and to select historical examples to buttress their opinions. And, finally, the regulations required all contestants to evaluate the political tendencies and parties in Germany ("from the revolutionary movements, on the one hand, to those of stagnation or reaction on the other") from the standpoint of their compatibility with the teachings of Darwin's theory of descent. All entries were expected to demonstrate "scientific merit" while simultaneously avoiding unnecessary technical jargon so as to be accessible to a lay audience. Although the contest was not limited to Germans, all manuscripts had to be presented in German.[19]

From all available sources we cannot say for certain whether Krupp himself actually handpicked those who, in addition to Haeckel and Ziegler, were to serve as judges for the contest. It seems reasonable to assume, however, that all of them were, if not openly sympathetic to Krupp's political conservatism, at least no friend of Germany's Social Democratic party. Fritz Krupp, as staunch an opponent of socialism as his father, could hardly have allowed sympathizers of Bebel to have the last word on the new biology—especially considering that he himself was paying to have the word spread. A brief look at the background of some of the judges supports this assumption.

All entries were examined by two different panels. The first *Schiedsgericht* (panel of judges) was composed of three respected scholars: Ziegler, zoologist; Johannes Conrad (1839–1915), economist; and Dietrich Schäfer (1845–1929), historian. These three men, representing three diverse and relevant fields, independently judged and ranked all manuscripts. A prize committee consisting of Haeckel, Conrad, and a Stuttgart geologist and paleontologist, Eberhard Fraas (1862–1915), was also established to settle any disparities and deadlocks among the three judges as to which entries merited a prize, and exactly which prize they deserved. The prize committee not only acted as final arbiter in the absence of a unanimous decision regarding the rank order of a particular manuscript but also communicated the official announcement of the judges' decision to the contestants.[20]

Of the three judges who made up the Schiedsgericht, two are known to have harbored conservative political views. Ziegler, probably the most influential man on the panel and a personal acquaintance of Krupp, made no secret of his disgust for Social Democracy. A dedicated student of August Weismann in Freiburg,[21] Ziegler was convinced that both the recent findings of his teacher on the subject of heredity, and Weismann's reinterpretation of Darwinian evolution, effectively eliminated the possibility of environmental factors playing a role in the evolutionary development of the human race. Since socialist theorists such as Bebel argued for the compatibility of Darwinism and socialism on the false assumption that a new environment (in the case of humans, a new form of society) would create a new species of humans, Ziegler felt compelled to set the story straight once and for all in a work entitled, *Die Naturwissenschaft und die socialdemokratische Theorie* (Science and Social Democratic Theory).[22] This work, allegedly an objective comparison of the views of Darwin and Bebel (as representatives of science and Social Democracy respectively), was actually an example of nascent scientism—in this case, an attempt to legitimize the political status quo by using science (biology) to discredit the efficacy and desirability of socialism. The zoologist's political sympathies were certainly close to those of the National Liberals—the party of big business.[23] Clearly, Ziegler was, from Krupp's point of view, an acceptable judge. The second judge, Johannes Conrad, was a member of the National Liberal party until that party's shift to protectionism in the 1880s.[24] The political leanings of the third member of the panel, Fraas, are unknown, although his position as curator of a royal scientific institution in Stuttgart precluded his holding any radical political opinions. Whether the judges were actually selected by Krupp or not, all had the appropriate credentials for the job.

The Krupp competition was announced by the members of the prize committee on January 1, 1900. Interested parties had until December 1, 1902 to submit their entries. In the period between the announcement and the final deadline for manuscripts, no less than sixty contestants formally entered the competition: forty-four from Germany, eight from Austria, four from Switzerland, and two each from the United States and Russia.[25] Of the original sixty, as Ziegler tells us, the panel of judges immediately disqualified fifteen entries for misinterpreting the question, being too short or otherwise insignificant, or propagating "very strange views" written in a totally inappropriate style.[26] Most of the remaining forty-five works, while differing widely in emphasis and intellectual orientation, could best be described as a heterogeneous collection of social Darwinist tracts.

The political tendencies of the entries and the ideological convictions of the authors indeed reflected virtually the entire spectrum of political opinion in turn-of-the-century Wilhelmine Germany, with the exception of the Catholic Center party. In his analysis of the results of the competition, Ziegler grouped Germany's political parties not into the traditional divisions of right and left but rather arranged them according to the degree to which the state was expected to intervene and carry out ascribed functions in society. According to this division there was only one contestant representing the extreme right, anarchy, and only a few "insignificant" authors defending Marxist socialism.[27] Several manuscripts demonstrated greatest sympathy with what Ziegler conveniently but most inappropriately designated as the "middle parties"—the National Liberals and Free Conservatives.[28] These works, he claimed, could not be characterized as being guided by great principles; rather, authors of Bismarck's political persuasion evaluated "each prospective law according to its practical usefulness for the individual and the society as a whole."[29] For the position of classical liberalism of the kind articulated by Herbert Spencer, Ziegler was able to claim but a single representative out of dozens of contestants. This one tract was the only work to "principally defend the old ideal of liberalism of direct universal suffrage, which is now in operation in the Reich" (at best a half truth considering its limitation to Reichstag elections). Many of the other entries proposed changes in the suffrage laws. This, according to Ziegler, suggested "that in educated circles the ideal [direct universal suffrage] has lost much of its old magic since its implementation."[30]

Although Darwin's theory of natural selection could best be linked to some sort of liberalism, most of the entries did not mirror the views of the celebrated English apologist of strict laissez-faire capitalism. As Ziegler himself recognized, the times were no longer ripe for liberalism.

> It is striking that the liberal view found expression merely in the above-mentioned treatise. This is all the more the case since it [liberalism] so easily lends itself to the principles of the theory of selec-

tion. I believe this can only be explained if one recognizes that in our day the general tendency points in another direction. Our times wish an increasing amount of social legislation, and this is possible only in the company of a strong state which, in the interest of the good of all, both dares to limit the freedom of the individual and regulates economic processes.[31]

In the aftermath of economic recession, Germany's turn to protectionism, and Bismarck's social legislation, liberalism, never very strong in Germany, was largely discredited. Reflecting the general shift in social and economic philosophy, approximately one-third of all entries advocated some form of state socialism as the alleged "political" consequence of an accurate interpretation of Darwinian evolution.[32] As we have seen, in Germany state socialism was by no means a radical philosophy.

On March 7, 1903, the prize committee announced the winners of the competition. In addition to a first prize and two second prizes, there were also five lesser monetary awards, apparently made possible by an increase in the total amount of money allotted by the Krupp family for the contest.[33] All eight award-winning manuscripts were to be published both individually and as part of a series entitled: *Natur und Staat: Beiträge zur naturwissenschaftlichen Gesellschaftslehre* (Nature and State: Contributions Towards a Scientific Study of Society). Underwritten over a period of fifteen years by the prestigious Jena-based science publishing company Gustav Fischer Verlag, the original series was expanded to encompass not only seven of the award-winning essays but also three additional works, including a lengthy treatise by one of the judges, Heinrich Ziegler, with the title *Die Vererbungslehre in der Biologie und in der Soziologie* (Heredity in Biology and Sociology). The decision to publish manuscripts as part of a series almost certainly attracted a greater amount of attention to the theme of the contest and to the individual responses than would have been possible had the entries merely been printed without any obvious connection to one another. From all indications, the contest and the series *Natur und Staat* served well the purpose of Fritz Krupp and the judges to demonstrate that Darwin's theory neither "possessed the state-damaging character attributed to it by its opponents," nor in any way "destroyed morals." Darwinism was shown to be inimical to Social Democracy, and, although opposed to Christian morality, it could be said to lay the groundwork for a new ethics with "a scientific-sociological basis."[34]

THE WINNING ENTRY:
VERERBUNG UND AUSLESE

As Ziegler observed in his introduction to the series, the best manuscripts tended to come from authors who used the competition simply as a good opportunity to give more concrete expression to views and opinions which had preoccupied their minds for years. Indeed, Haeckel, Conrad, and Fraas awarded the first prize to a physician who, for at least fourteen years prior to his entry into the contest, had been deeply concerned with the political meaning of Darwin's theory of descent. Wilhelm Schallmayer's 381-page *Vererbung und Auslese* representing, as Ziegler appraised it, a "hygienic-sociological" approach to the question, attested to the author's long-standing commitment to the issues articulated in his first treatise.[35] But while his earlier, little-known work did little more than summarize in less than fifty pages the problem of degeneration and offer a few proposals to combat it, Schallmayer's award-winning essay not only placed "heredity" and "selection" in a greatly expanded historical and political framework, but also provided a wealth of detailed "evidence" demonstrating the connection between degeneration and the new biology. Schallmayer's work, which only later and in a revised edition became the standard German eugenics textbook, sought to prove that the real political lesson to be learned from Darwin's theory was that long-term state power depended on the biological vitality of the nation; any "mismanagement" of the hereditary fitness of its population, such as might result from unenlightened laws and customs, was "bad politics" and would inevitably result in the downfall of the state.[36] In the interest of self-preservation, argued the Bavarian physician, it was imperative that the state take an active part in regulating the overall biological efficiency of its citizens by embarking on a political program which would encourage the biologically best elements in society to reproduce more than those with objectionable hereditary traits.

In his treatise Schallmayer did, of course, have to address himself to the specific questions and guidelines laid out by Krupp and the prize committee for the purposes of the contest. All contestants were obligated to take a position on the question of heredity and the role of nonbiological factors in the evolution of society, as well as evaluate Germany's political parties with an eye toward their compatibility with the teachings of Darwin. It is both interesting and revealing to observe how Schallmayer, in an attempt to satisfy both the requirements of the contest and the demands inherent in his own thesis, was brilliantly able to weave biological, historical, and political "facts" into a convincing argument which the judges believed worthy to be taken with the utmost seriousness.

Schallmayer allotted two brief pages of the preface to set the proper historical framework for what was to follow. The nineteenth century, he suggested, was marked by great theoretical advances in the natural sciences. Towering above all other scientific achievements was the birth and "triumph" of Darwin's theory of organic evolution. Darwin's theory not only revolutionized many of the biological sciences but also threw new light on the social sciences. However, in contrast to the preceding century's preoccupation with scientific theories, the coming epoch was assigned a more challenging task. "The twentieth century," argued Schallmayer, "is called upon to apply the theory of descent to everyday life."[37] As he envisaged it, *Vererbung und Auslese* was to deal with the practical and political application of Darwinism.

Before Schallmayer could elaborate upon "practical applications" of the theory of descent, however, he had to first provide the reader with the necessary biological background. Schallmayer devoted the first chapter of his book to a discussion of evolutionary theory—with special emphasis, as one might expect, on Darwin's contribution. "As opposed to earlier opinions, Darwinian evolution or Darwinism," remarked Schallmayer, "is characterized by the principle of selection." Such a representation made it quite easy for Schallmayer to refer to Darwinian evolution as simply "the theory of selection"; the fact that Darwin himself incorporated principles other than natural selection to account for the transmutation of species was quite immaterial.[38]

> The principle of natural selection is what made evolutionary theory important. Previously it was only an interesting conjecture discussed, without more or less conviction, by various scholars and thinkers without finding a reception in wider circles. Only as a result of the union of the descent theory and the theory of selection did evolution become a force which, despite strong opposition, old prejudices and powerful interests, continues to pave new roads—a force which, despite contemporary assaults against it, will endure without injury.[39]

Taking the lead from Haeckel, a man who went far beyond Darwin in his willingness to explain "human nature" and human society solely as a result of the principle of selection, Schallmayer in a later chapter established natural selection as the precondition of all social progress—past, present, and future— and warned of the danger should it no longer remain effective.

> From Darwin's theory of selection it may undoubtedly be said that selection is the prerequisite for progress, and that the stronger the selection, the greater the progress. A further consequence of the theory is that progress is not just desirable, but at least in the long run, a necessity. From this necessity there is no escape—nor has there ever been since the beginning of life. Moreover, without the continuous [presence] of selection, even the level of development arrived at so far cannot be maintained.[40]

Once having fully identified Darwinism with the principle of selection, Schallmayer used the remainder of the first chapter to briefly acquaint his audience with the important assumptions of the theory. One of the four assumptions built into Darwinian evolution was the idea that variations existing among organisms in a population would be inherited by future generations. Yet the critical question of the mechanism of heredity remained unsolved and indeed largely unasked during Darwin's lifetime. Darwin himself, realizing the importance of explaining inheritance, sought to remedy the situation by adopting a theory of pangenesis. Even before his death however, most biologists recognized the gross inadequacies of Darwin's explanation, although they themselves were unable to provide a viable alternative. In his first treatise Schallmayer had lamented the fact that so little was known about such an important subject.

Sometime between 1895 and 1900, Schallmayer found in the work of August Weismann the scientific study of heredity he had long sought. Not only did Weismann's views on heredity reflect and reinforce the "selectionist" emphasis given to Darwin's theory of descent in the 1890s but also appeared to Schallmayer to be more sophisticated, more exact, and more scientific than any of the numerous competing Lamarckian theories. For Schallmayer it was Weismann "who first provided us with the key to understanding the hereditary process."[41] Yet this was of course the biased assumption of an individual who was committed to Weismann's work largely for nonbiological reasons. His "discovery" of Weismann may have spelled the end of his own imprecisely defined Lamarckian outlook, but his reasons for choosing Weismann during the heyday of Neo-Lamarckism were largely self-serving.[42] Unlike several Anglo-American eugenicists, most notably Charles Davenport, Schallmayer had little or no training in biology beyond the medically related subjects of anatomy and physiology.[43] Given his lack of expertise, he was not in the position to make a scientifically informed decision on the relative merits of the competing hereditary theories. The rules of the contest, however, did require Schallmayer to take a stand. He expressed his immense admiration for the works of Weismann by devoting over forty pages of *Verbung und Auslese* to an explanation of the Freiburg zoologist's biological theories, especially the "continuity of the germ-plasm." Since the rediscovery of Mendel's work only occurred in 1900—the year the contest was announced—it is not surprising that it was not mentioned in Schallmayer's treatise. Subsequent editions of *Vererbung and Auslese*, however, did include a discussion of Mendel's theory of heredity. Yet like his devotion to Weismann's work, Schallmayer's favorable reception of Mendelism does not account for his turn to eugenics—it served to legitimize it.

Schallmayer began his elaboration of the science of heredity by explaining the process of meiosis (reproduction of sex cells) to his readers, using diagrams taken from Weismann's most mature work, *Vorträge über Descendenztheorie* (Lectures on the Theory of Descent). After a lengthy description of the components of Weismann's germ-plasm (that is, biophores, determinants, ids, and idents) and how changes in its material composition resulted in the creation of a new species through a continuous selection of fortuitous variations in the hereditary substance, Schallmayer stated his unequivocal opposition to the inheritance of acquired characteristics. So-called Lamarckian environmental influences played no role in the transmutation of species. Selection alone, acting upon what Weismann terms "plus or minus variations" found in all organisms, was sufficient to account for the evolutionary process.[44]

Having taken the required stand on the question of heredity, Schallmayer went still further and attempted to use the language and theories of Weismann to render plausible his fear of biological degeneration. He affirmed the efficacy of Weismann's Panmixie as an explanation of why organs degenerate, and cited a previously quoted passage on birds of prey (see chapter 1) to demonstrate that the elimination of natural selection must inevitably lead to the degeneration of animal and human races—possibly to their extinction. He also accepted Weismann's account of why an increasing number of people were in need of glasses.[45] And finally, Weismann's theory of germinal selection was able to adequately render intelligible for Schallmayer the "conspicuous appearance of the progressive degeneration of psychopathically tainted families, which until now lacked a viable explanation."[46]

Schallmayer also used Weismann's theories to sanction a new code of ethics—a "generative ethics." In his 1882 essay, *On the Duration of Life*, Weismann had discussed the relationship between the individual and the species. According to Weismann, the average length of life of an individual is governed by the needs of the species to which it belonged. From the standpoint of the species, once the individual reproduced itself it was no longer important; it "has performed its share of this work of compensation, it ceases to be of any value to the species, it has fulfilled its duties and may die."[47] Weismann's message was clear: individuals exist to serve a larger unit; their existence is justified insofar as they complete their task of reproduction.

Schallmayer sought to extract the ethical lessons of Weismann's biology. He never tired of repudiating the Benthamite pleasure principle with its individualism and its emphasis upon the happiness of the present-day generation. Such an ethical system could never be in agreement with evolutionary theory.[48] For Schallmayer, biology clearly demonstrated that all human feelings and desires were merely selective adaptive traits which insured that the individual carried out its reproductive functions.

We cannot avoid observing that in nature, the interest of the individual is subordinate to that of the species. It appears as if the individual exists only to perform a function for the species and is not an end in itself; individuals no longer of worth to the maintenance of the species are blessed with an early death. As Weismann had demonstrated, the duration of life of every species is regulated to fit its needs. . . . Death itself is, according to Weismann, a service to the species at the expense of the individuals. This law of nature, the total subservience of the interest of the individual to that of the species, must also hold true for human development.[49]

Weismann's views thus had practical implications for politics and ethics. Just as the interest of the individual should not take precedence over that of the species, politics should not further the interest of contemporary society at the expense of the nation's future. Ethics must be concerned with the preservation of society and, hence, must be designed to further the biological vitality of the nation. Clearly a "generative" or "evolutionary" ethics was needed in the day-to-day politics of Germany. The new biology, while destroying outdated moral codes based on both the teachings of Christ and possessive individualism, also laid the foundation for a new scientifically based ethical imperative: the biological efficiency of the state.

The controversy surrounding the inheritance of acquired characteristics would hardly have received such widespread attention (and hence become an issue of the Krupp contest) had not everyone agreed on the importance of heredity. The psychiatric and neurological establishment labeled an innumerable number of asocial traits "pathological" and then demonstrated how they were transmitted from one generation to the next in accordance with the laws of inheritance. In this Schallmayer was no exception; he devoted several pages of *Vererbung und Auslese* to a discussion of the inheritance of pathological traits and their negative impact.[50] But pathological or "defective" traits were not the only characteristics recognized by Schallmayer as following the dictates of heredity. Following the lead of Darwin, he argued for the transmission of a large number of physical traits as well as numerous so-called instincts (e.g., self-preservation, reproductive drive, altruism, compassion, etc.). But, more important, Schallmayer, citing the recent work of Francis Galton on the subject, championed the inheritance of "mental traits."[51] This extremely vague and general term was understood by Schallmayer to mean everything from moral qualities to intelligence.

The importance Schallmayer attributed to heredity in the evolutionary process was matched only by his belief in the efficacy of natural selection. The principle of selection insured that the most favorable traits survived; heredity saw to it that such traits were preserved over time. Collectively these two factors accounted for the enormous organic and social progress visible on the globe. Schallmayer's decision to champion Weismann in the ongoing debate over heredity was directly related both to the Freiburg zoologist's ability to provide a mechanism of inheritance as well as his insistence on the *Allmacht* (omnipotence) of natural selection.

As critical as the selection of desirable physical and mental traits was for the progress of social evolution, it alone did not tell the entire story. Responding to the prize committee's request that all contestants evaluate the role of nonbiological factors in the rise and fall of states and civilizations, Schallmayer devoted a large portion of his book to the relative importance of tradition, customs, and institutions as significant variables in the development of human society. Culture-specific practices and achievements such as sexual mores, family structure, modes of production, organized religion, technology, and legal codes were, according to Schallmayer, also subject to the iron law of selection, albeit indirectly. Those customs and institutions which afforded its practitioners a competitive edge in the struggle for survival among nations and states were selected insofar as the individuals practicing them survived at the expense of other people less well equipped. Cultural practices which did not enhance the fitness of the tribe or nation disappeared with the extinction of those individuals comprising that political unit; customs and institutions of proven ability in the struggle for survival were passed on to future generations and tended to remain in effect as long as they promoted the overall efficiency of those practicing them.[52] Schallmayer singled out monogamy as one example of a successful age-old cultural practice. Clearly, without the strong familial ties effected by monogamous relationships, society would not have inched beyond the level reached by Africa's and Australia's most primitive tribes.

For Schallmayer, both history and contemporary society were replete with examples of how accepted cultural practices determined the fate of nations and civilizations. Citing the work of Otto Seeck, a nineteenth-century historian of the ancient world,[53] Schallmayer sought to demonstrate that a shift in ethical values away from marriage and raising children resulted in the eventual decline of Greece and Rome. The widespread use of prostitutes by Roman patricians was said by Schallmayer to have lowered the value of women as objects of desire and resulted in a rapid increase in homosexuality;[54] a declining fertility rate, especially among the most biologically desirable Roman classes, inevitably resulted in Rome's inability to defend itself against attacks by the barbarian hordes. China, in contrast, with its large families, strong kinship ties, aristocracy of talent rather than birth, absence of primogeniture, and so forth, was testimony to the extraordinary old age a civilization could reach with the aid of population-promoting institutions and practices.[55] Unlike many European intellectuals who asserted the physical, intellectual, and cultural inferiority of the Chinese to the "white race," Schallmayer praised the exemplary hereditary traits of that ancient people and the high biological worth of their customs—going even so far as to argue, in a later tract, that they had a larger average cranial capacity than the Germans![56]

Although the precise origins of Schallmayer's complementary attitude toward the Chinese are unknown, his experience in 1894 as ship's physician on board a German vessel traveling to the Far East certainly played a part in shaping it. Whether his extensive reading of Chinese cultural history served merely to confirm his personal impression of the Chinese workers he met aboard his ship or, what seems more likely, his brief acquaintance with the Chinese solidified the prejudices acquired through book learning, Schallmayer's trip made a lasting impression on him. Throughout his life he continued to uphold China as a perfect example of a society whose culture promoted rather than curtailed the long-term survival and vitality of a people; Schallmayer hoped that his own country would take a few lessons from the Chinese.[57]

After this extended discussion of the biological and historical impact of heredity and selection on both nature and human society, Schallmayer returned to the central question of the competition: what does Darwinian evolution teach us about internal political development and state legislation? For the author the answer was clear. Just as the preservation of the species was the goal of biological development, so too must the preservation of the state become the "end" of politics. In order to maintain itself in the competitive struggle among nations, the state must shape its politics such that the "greatest possible increase of power" is guaranteed. "[T]he highest aim of domestic politics, to which all other goals are subservient, is to shape the conditions for existence within the population as dictated by the need for power necessary for the international struggle for survival."[58]

How, then, could the state work toward the one "scientific" goal of all political development: national preservation? First, state power presupposed a thoroughgoing rationalization of human society. Political power was no longer simply a function of how quickly a nation could mobilize its armed forces for combat. Indeed, the military might of a state largely depended on its level of economic and technical efficiency. As Schallmayer put it, power presupposed both an "ever-increasing division of labor" and a "continuous decrease in the squandering of manpower." Moreover, improved organization would raise the *Nutzeffekt* (efficiency) of individual as well as collective productivity.[59] Only state socialism, Schallmayer believed, could achieve the requisite level of efficiency; the chaos of unbridled laissez-faire capitalism could not.

But economic rationalization, although necessary for national efficiency, was hardly the entire solution. A form of population management was also a political imperative. State power was the result of a quantitatively large and qualitatively healthy population, and statesmen must formulate national policy with this view in mind.

Since a large population is an essential element of power and a prerequisite for a higher development of social organization, all efforts in the area of domestic as well as foreign policy must be judged from the standpoint of whether they are likely to strengthen or weaken the ability of the population to *survive* and *procreate*. . . . However, it is not simply a matter of the quantity of population, but also a question of the population's *social productivity [soziale Leistungsfähigkeit]*. . . . in order for the state to hold its own or have supremacy over the other peoples, domestic policy must not neglect the hereditary composition of the population. *Future political development will prove more successful the more it secures the effectiveness of a generative selection*—a selection which is not only the necessary condition for all progress but even for the preservation of the status quo.[60]

Thus, it was necessary for the state not only to rationally manage its economy but also its population. Here again Schallmayer uses an economic analogy: the relationship between state and society, he contended, is the same as that between "the landowner and his tenants"; that is, the state must encourage the populace not to squander its labor and procreative power for short-term gain, but rather to administer them for the long-term good of society.[61]

Measured by these standards, none of Germany's political parties were truly biologically informed. Each one failed to extract the "correct" political meaning from Darwin's theory of descent and adjust its party program and platform accordingly. Had Fritz Krupp been alive when the results of the contest were finally announced, he would have most certainly been disappointed with the views and opinions articulated in Schallmayer's essay.[62] Schallmayer was not the least bit sympathetic to the profit-and-influence-seeking philosophy of the House of Krupp, and in fact only agreed to enter the contest after written assurance by Haeckel that all entries would be judged solely on the basis of "scientific merit," without regard to the contestant's personal political convictions.[63] From Schallmayer's point of view, the Free Conservatives and National Liberals, the parties most representative of Krupp's political leanings, were like all other German parties: nothing more than highly organized special-interest lobbies that had long ago abandoned any claim of serving the welfare of the entire nation. At a time when Germany's political parties were little more than weak and dogmatic representatives of single class or group interests, Schallmayer, like many German intellectuals, placed his faith in some form of extraparliamentary movement which could transcend class differences and party distinctions.[64] For Schallmayer, eugenics alone held open the promise of becoming a movement above the parties and capable of bringing together all individuals who truly had the national interest at heart.

While Schallmayer distanced himself from all of Germany's political parties, he did, as was mentioned previously, have "socialist leanings." His state socialist sympathies, however, did not lead to his endorsement of the Social Democratic party and its platform. Although he praised the Social Democrats for the positive support of science education in the schools and their position regarding collective ownership of the means of production, Schallmayer attacked the Marxists for their one-sided preoccupation with economics and working-class interests as well as for their goal of economic equality for all.[65]

About the last point he was particularly uncompromising. Like most eugenicists, Schallmayer proceeded from the assumption that individuals are not biologically equal. Since a person's social productivity and social usefulness were largely a product of his or her "biological fitness," any attempt to institute the communist maxim "from each according to his abilities, to each according to his needs" would not only penalize the most enterprising members of society but would also tip the scales in favor of the genetically least-suited citizens and hence promote degeneration. According to Schallmayer, "the most desirable distribution of wealth was one which best promoted social productivity as well as provided the best incentive for the biologically fit to reproduce."[66] Quoting the German economist Gustav Schmoller on the functional importance of retaining the Protestant work ethic, Schallmayer affirmed the necessity of classes and the social and economic rewards afforded by class mobility as a means of insuring ever-higher levels of national economic productivity.[67] But even assuming it were possible to forcibly eliminate classes in the construction of a utopian socialist society, new "natural" classes would soon be formed based on individual differences in performance. Schallmayer's political ideal was a *Leistungsaristokratie* (meritocracy), whereby the most advanced form of human and economic organization, a form of state socialism, would be created in order to promote a higher level of national efficiency. His meritocratic outlook was remarkably akin to that of his future British colleague Karl Pearson.[68]

Having established that none of Germany's political parties was truly compatible with the teachings of Darwin, Schallmayer presented his readers with a series of reforms touching numerous social, political, and economic institutions in an attempt to "prepare the nation for the struggle for survival." Included among his suggestions were some already discussed in his first treatise (e.g., tax on the military unfit, the creation of family genealogies, promotion of research in the area of heredity), as well as a few ideas that were only implicitly entertained in his earlier essay. Although Schallmayer did not present a clearly articulated list of eugenic proposals in the first edition of *Vererbung und Auslese*, his disparate statements on the subject can, for the sake of convenience, be categorized under the following headings: negative eugenics, positive eugenics, and public hygiene.[69]

Included under the rubric of negative eugenics were all measures, both voluntary and involuntary, direct and indirect, which sought to prevent or at least strongly discourage the "unfit" and "defective" from reproducing. Returning once again to the militarily unfit, Schallmayer suggested that those men rejected for military duty be discouraged from marrying at an earlier age than that of the average conscript, who had to wait until after the completion of his service.[70] He was also favorably inclined toward either sterilizing proven hereditary criminals in order to protect society from generations of lawbreakers, or permanently placing them in a criminal asylum, an idea advocated by London's retired chief of police. The latter remedy would not only lessen the burden of the courts and protect society from such morally defective individuals but also would alleviate the constant state of tension experienced by the criminal as he tries in vain to suppress his hereditary tendency toward crime in order to avoid punishment.[71]

On the whole, however, Schallmayer proceeded with the utmost caution in the area of negative eugenics. In doing so he helped shape the emphasis upon voluntary measures among German race hygienists—a tradition also particularly strong in Britain.[72] Although he clearly believed that marriage restrictions for the insane, the feeble-minded, the chronic alcoholic, the hereditary criminal, the tubercular, and those not fully cured of venereal disease were in the best interests of national efficiency, Schallmayer refrained from openly supporting state legislation as a means to this end. Until such time as more exact information regarding the laws of heredity was known and until enough detailed hereditary genealogies could be amassed, those interested in the welfare of the nation would have to concentrate their efforts on voluntary measures. In Schallmayer's opinion much could be accomplished by instituting and developing a new moral code—a more polite way of suggesting that through propaganda and indoctrination people would eventually be made to recognize the danger of an unbridled increase in the "unfit." In the long run, Schallmayer hoped, a new generative ethics would result in a decline in the number of dysgenic marriages on the part of those rational enough to adhere to scientific testimony, and would pave the way for future legislative action by mobilizing popular support for eugenics.

"Generative ethics" were not only an important element of negative eugenics but also played a major role in what Schallmayer considered the more significant side of his overall strategy: positive eugenics. Here too Schallmayer set a trend visible in the subsequent history of the pre-Nazi German race hygiene movement. Schallmayer defined as positive eugenics all measures (both voluntary and involuntary) which encouraged the "fitter" groups and classes of society to increase their fertility rate. The question of course remained: which national groups and classes are, biologically speaking, the "fittest"? Schallmayer hoped that eventually the "science of heredity" would settle the issue in an objective, scientific manner. Until this new biological discipline reached maturity, however, relative fitness would be determined by a group's overall contribution to society. "In the meantime," argued Schallmayer, "it would not be incorrect to view highly socially productive individuals, especially the better educated, as being, on the average, more biologically valuable."[73] As Schallmayer saw it, "high-ranking civil servants, including officers and teachers, should remain single as infrequently as possible and marry as early as possible." Those who chose to remain single should suffer some sort of financial disadvantage. To encourage high-level civil servants to have larger families, Schallmayer suggested that they be given a bonus for each school-age child.[74] The class bias implicit in Schallmayer's criteria regarding "fitness" could hardly be more blatant; the biologically "fit" turn out to be individuals from the same socioeconomic group as Schallmayer: the educated middle classes.

Schallmayer envisaged that the measures and proposals here categorized under the heading of negative and positive eugenics would form a new branch of hygiene which he labeled *Vererbungshygiene* (hereditary hygiene).[75] The Germanized term *Eugenik* was not used by the author until 1907. Indeed, by the time of publication of *Vererbung und Auslese*, Schallmayer had already investigated eugenics-related proposals and legislation outside of Germany; he was particularly impressed by attempts in America to put eugenics into practice.[76]

Yet eugenics, albeit the most important branch of hygiene from the standpoint of national efficiency was not the only one. The third and final part of his program to promote the long-term health of the nation included measures that fall under the general category of social and public hygiene. His campaign to educate and safeguard against alcoholism and venereal disease deserves particular attention. Schallmayer actively supported steps taken by the American and Swedish temperance unions in their attempt to combat alcohol consumption, contrasting such efforts with the *Trinkpoesie* (glorification of alcohol) of his own country.[77] The fight against intoxication and alcoholism was particularly important because alcohol was generally believed by physicians at the time to adversely affect a person's germ-plasm, or hereditary material, and therefore contributed to degeneration. Schallmayer also warmly welcomed the establishment of the German Society for the Fight Against Venereal Disease and reiterated earlier proposals from his first treatise to combat the spread of syphilis and gonorrhea, and to warn against their long-term degenerative effects.[78]

Schallmayer's disparate proposals to help boost national efficiency were stimulated by the specific requirements demanded of all Krupp competition contestants. His views became widely known in both German academic and medical circles as a result of the publication of his *Vererbung und Auslese* as part of the series *Natur und Staat*. The reaction to Schallmayer's book, however, was by no means universally favorable. Not only were Schallmayer's suggestions and views of political reality regarded by many as both bizarre and novel but they also tended to alienate individuals who felt professionally threatened by Schallmayer's intrusion onto their academic turf. In the course of the next fifteen years, Schallmayer fought with various academic elites and special-interest groups over the disciplinary integrity of eugenics and the efficacy of *Rassehygiene* as a means of solving the social question. The result of this continuous dialogue between Schallmayer and representatives of other disciplines was the crystallization, elaboration, and further popularization of Schallmayer's eugenic thought.

IV

CONTINUITY AND CONTROVERSY: SCHALLMAYER'S DEFENSE OF EUGENICS

During the three years immediately following the publication of *Vererbung und Auslese* in 1903, Schallmayer's book was reviewed in at least two newspapers and over twenty literary and academic journals, ranging from philosophy to medicine and spanning the political spectrum from arch-conservatism to socialism. Later editions of his treatise (1910 and 1918), as well as Schallmayer's third work, *Beiträge zu einer Nationalbiologie* (Contributions to a National Biology) (1905), continued to attract attention in a large number of professional publications.[1] Although *Vererbung und Auslese* was not without its wholehearted admirers, the critical reviews of the text far outweighed the complimentary. Indeed, given the aim and scope of the work, the unfavorable reception it received in many circles was a foregone conclusion. In attempting as it did to redefine and reexamine old social, political, and medical problems from a new, allegedly "scientific" perspective, Schallmayer's treatise cut across several well-entrenched disciplinary boundaries. It is not surprising that Schallmayer's intentional breach of academic territoriality, together with the perceived inadequacies of his intellectual premises, alarmed and often angered practitioners of the disciplines in question. Even after a decade of sustained clarification of the assumptions and aims of eugenics, and after years of assurances on the part of Schallmayer that eugenics did not seek to put the more traditional disciplines out of business, many individuals continued to attack the intellectual hubris and professional pretensions of the upstart field and its spokesmen.

Of the interest groups and academic elites who took offense at the claims of Schallmayer and other eugenicists, the "social anthropologists,"[2] social scientists, and public hygienists stand out as the most vocal. The verbal assaults directed at *Vererbung und Auslese* by representatives of these three groups initiated a series of heated intellectual controversies with Schallmayer which never fully abated. Although not without interest in their own right, these controversies become particularly important when examined from the standpoint of the development and maturation of Schallmayer's view on race hygiene. The eugenicist's dispute with the three groups highlight three fundamental tenets of Schallmayer's eugenic thought: first, that eugenics has nothing to do with ideologies of Aryan or Nordic supremacy; second, that the goal of biological efficiency necessitates a biologically informed sociology as well as the reconstruction and reformulation of German social policy; and third, that eugenics is an extension, not a replacement, of traditional public hygiene. Despite differences in immediate goals, both eugenics and public hygiene were part of a larger, three-part program to promote Germany's biological fitness which Schallmayer labeled *biologische Politik* (biological policy).

Notwithstanding his increasingly heavy emphasis after 1908 on the third part of his program, "quantitative population policy," Schallmayer's views exhibit an unusual degree of intellectual cohesion and continuity. His overriding objective from beginning to end was to increase the hereditary efficiency of the nation; all his plans, programs, and schema, varied as they were, were directed toward the attainment of this one goal. Schallmayer's controversies with the social anthropologists, social scientists, and public hygienists at once reveal this continuity of vision and some of the obstacles preventing its realization.

RACE HYGIENE AGAINST RACISM

Of all the critiques directed against Schallmayer's text, none was as polemical, petty, and self-serving as those made by the so-called German school of *Sozialanthropologie* (social anthropology)—a movement which developed parallel to eugenics, but one that, at least until the Nazi period, was not really part of race hygiene.[3] While social anthropology had many affinities to eugenics (largely owing to the set of social Darwinist assumptions held in common), it was regarded as an independent discipline by its practitioners and fellow travelers, complete with its own methodologies, objectives, and journal. The major thrust of this discipline was to provide a scientific legitimation for ideologies of Aryan supremacy. Though individual Nordic enthusiasts were found among the eugenicists, this movement fell outside the mainstream of Wilhelmine eugenics.

The intellectual origins of social anthropology can be traced to the writings and influence of the French diplomat, publicist, and aristocrat Comte Arthur de Gobineau (1816 – 1882).[4] Best known for his lengthy two-volume *Essai sur l'Inégalité des Races Humaines* (Essay on the Inequality of Human Races) (1853 – 55), Gobineau was above all obsessed with the question of why civilizations have declined in the past and why contemporary civilizations are destined for decay in the future.[5] Gobineau, whose pessimistic view of the historical process was colored by his inability to accept the political realities of postrevolutionary France, believed he had found the key to the inevitable decline of civilizations in a single factor: racial mixture. Each of the three so-called major races—white, yellow, and black—possessed, according to Gobineau, their own particular virtues and characteristics. These racial traits accounted for the cultural diversity of past and present civilizations. The catch, of course, was that the races were not only different but also unequal. For Gobineau the white race, or "Aryans,"[6] embraced the lofty ideals of freedom, honor, and spirituality—the virtues that, as George Mosse has aptly pointed out, corresponded to his vision of the French nobility.[7] Moreover, only the white race (which itself could be divided into several subraces, with the Nordic or Germanic representing the pinnacle of Aryan virtue) was capable of creating a truly great civilization. The yellow and black races, while not totally lacking in favorable traits, were decidedly inferior to the white race and were equated, in the mind of Gobineau, with the bourgeoisie and the proletariat respectively.[8]

As Gobineau viewed it, civilizations began to decline when the races or subraces which engendered them mixed with other inferior races, thus polluting the racial composition of the indigenous population. The process of racial hybridization, with its ominous results for the Germanic subrace and those nations founded upon it, was inescapable. In the past, people of different races always migrated to new lands and intermarried with the native people of the region. All evidence suggested that they will continue to do so. Gobineau thus resigned himself to the inevitable "degeneration" of the so-called Aryan race and the allegedly superior culture that only it made possible.[9]

Gobineau's philosophy of Aryan supremacy and his emphasis on race as the motive force of world history never gained much of a foothold in his native France; Germany proved to be far more intellectually receptive to his ideas. Through his personal friendship with the composer Richard Wagner, Gobineau's name became well-known among members of the conservative, anti-Semitic Bayreuth circle.[10] In 1894 the librarian and publicist Ludwig Schemann (1852–1938), an influential member of the Bayreuth circle, founded a Gobineau society. As a result of Schemann's efforts, Gobineau's racism reached numerous right-wing groups, the most important of which was the militaristic, anti-Semitic Pan-German League.[11] During the next forty years, Gobineau's ideas were extended and modified to fit the specifications of the völkisch right until they found their way, admittedly in a grossly distorted guise, into National Socialist ideology.

Gobineau's *Essai*, which was published before Darwin's *Origin of Species*, rested primarily on second-hand historical and linguistic "evidence"; the French aristocrat never attempted to

incorporate biological or anthropological theories into his philosophy of history. Some of his followers, however, had a broader perspective. By combining the selectionism of the Weismann-
ists, the craniometric techniques developed by the French
school of physical anthropology, and the culturally and lin-
guistically based racism of Gobineau, a younger generation of
Gobineau admirers created a new brand of racism that, at least in
some circles, enjoyed an aura of scientific respectability. In Germany, this venomous intellectual concoction went by the name
"social anthropology." It enjoyed some measure of popularity
from roughly the late 1880s until World War I.[12]

The three social anthropologists most actively engaged in intellectual battle with Schallmayer were also the three main theoretical spokesmen for their field. Perhaps the most articulate
among them, although not the most important from the standpoint of the subsequent debate, was the French librarian and
university lecturer Georges Vacher de Lapouge (1854–1936).[13]
Like Gobineau, Lapouge was held in much higher regard on the
right bank of the Rhine than on the left. Kaiser Wilhelm II championed him as "the only great Frenchman."[14] In fact by 1900,
Lapouge's writings, ridiculed in France, were published mainly
in Germany. By the turn of the century, the French social anthropologist had developed close intellectual ties with his German colleagues; indeed during his lifetime Lapouge contributed
about sixty articles to the *Politisch-anthropologische Revue* (Politi-
cal-Anthropological Review), the professional journal of the
German Gobineau school.

Stripped to its bare essentials, Lapouge's views can be summarized as follows: the "Aryan race" is the only race capable of
high social, intellectual, and cultural achievements, and is in fact
the true biological underpinning of Western civilization. The
Aryans, recognizable by a constellation of physical traits including blue eyes, blond hair, and, most important, a long oval-
shaped (dolichocephalic) head, were at the losing end of a constant Darwinian struggle of survival with inferior stock—in particular, with the brown-eyed, brown-haired, round-headed

"brachycephalic race."[15] The disastrous effects of this racial struggle could already be observed in France, where the once common Aryan had become an endangered species at the expense of an ever-growing proportion of other racial types. Since in addition to physical differences all races possessed their own unique intellectual, psychological, and even political characteristics, the West (and France in particular), was in danger of a great increase in the aesthetically unappealing larger average cephalic index. Because different social classes have demonstrably different racial compositions (the higher classes containing more pure Aryan types), Occidental civilization stood at the threshold of a degenerate era when non-Aryan bourgeois or even proletarian arrangements would displace Aryan aristocratic privilege and power. In short, the goal of social anthropology was to examine empirically the life process of the "Aryan race"—to describe its social and geographical diffusion, to evaluate the effects of selective and counterselective factors for its long-term survival, and finally, to propose measures that would restore the predominance of the Aryans.[16]

Lapouge's presuppositions and disciplinary program, if not his extreme pessimism, were echoed in the work of his German colleague, Otto Ammon (1862–1916). Like Lapouge, Ammon assumed that there was a direct correlation between hereditary fitness and social standing—a class bias Schallmayer shared, albeit in a much less blatant and exaggerated form. Ammon used the opinions and language of Weismann and Galton to support his claim that the various social classes represented a necessary form of natural selection, and should be preserved intact at all costs. Indeed, his defense of a meritocratic social order would seem to assure his good standing with many German eugenicists, particularly with Schallmayer.[17] Yet Ammon, following Lapouge, never failed to link biological fitness and high social standing with Nordic or Germanic stock, and was primarily concerned with demonstrating a correlation between class and racial composition. Using so-called objective statistical evidence from army recruits in the southwest German state of Baden, Ammon not only "proved" that the higher classes contained a larger percentage of dolichocephalic Nordic types,[18] but also that "city dwellers have a higher proportion of long-headed [individuals] among them than do those from the countryside."[19] Ammon was convinced that the larger Nordic element among city dwellers could be explained by the fact that individuals of Germanic stock, who possessed a "somewhat higher drive toward achievement,"[20] found little chance for material advancement in the countryside and hence often migrated to the towns. Ammon's one-sided preoccupation with the Aryan question far overshadowed the presuppositions and goals he held in common with Schallmayer.

The third, and from the standpoint of the ensuing controversy most important social anthropologist, was the zoologist and physician Ludwig Woltmann (1871–1907).[21] A one-time member of the German Social Democratic party, Woltmann began his intellectual career with an attempt to synthesize historical materialism, Darwinism and neo-Kantianism.[22] By 1900, however, Woltmann had more or less abandoned his utopian synthesis and turned his attention from " the dialectics of class struggle. . . to the philosophy of race struggle."[23] Like Ammon and Lapouge, Woltmann placed the "Germanic race" at the pinnacle of human evolution, but unlike the other social anthropologists Woltmann used aesthetic rather than "anthropological/scientific" evidence to support his contention. For Woltmann, the Aryan embodied the ideal of physical and spiritual beauty—a beauty constantly compromised, as he kept reminding his readers, by dysgenic racial mixtures with non-Germanic stock. During the last years of his short life Woltmann published *Die Germanen und die Renaissance in Italien* (The Teutons and the Renaisance in Italy) (1905) in which he argued that outstanding men of the Italian Renaissance such as Dante and Michelangelo were descendants of the Germanic tribes, not the Romans.[24]

In addition to their books, the social anthropologists sought other means of communicating their ideas to a larger audience. All utilized the *Politisch-anthropologische Revue*, founded and financed by Woltmann, to popularize their goals and promote their new discipline. Woltmann himself published scores of articles in his journal, not always under his own name.[25] But even prior to the founding of the *Revue* in 1902, Woltmann and Ammon attempted to publicize their views by entering the Krupp competition—an endeavor that met with mixed results.

It was disapppointing but not devastating for Ammon to learn that the third edition of his treatise, *Die Gesellschaftsordnung und ihre natürlichen Grundlagen* (The Social Order and Its Natural Foundations) (1900) did not receive a prize; after all the rules governing the contest specifically prohibited the judges from extending an award to books already published.[26] Woltmann, however, had a far more difficult time trying to rationalize the results of the competition. Woltmann's 326-page entry, *Politische Anthropologie* (Political Anthropology) only merited third prize— an honor which the German social anthropologist was asked to share with three other contestants.[27] Woltmann, insulted that the judges did not seem to share his own ridiculously high opinion of his text, refused to accept the award and began an extraordinarily nasty and petty campaign to discredit the contest, the judges, and above all, the contest's first prize winner.[28] The verbal attack launched by Woltmann against one of the judges reached such proportions that he was brought to court on a libel suit and fined three hundred marks.[29]

Insofar as Woltmann's critique of the two judges (Schäfer and Conrad) had any intellectual substance at all, it was directed against their alleged ignorance of the newest anthropological findings (meaning the work of the social anthropologists) and their seeming disregard for the importance of race in determining the contours of social evolution and human history. For Woltmann, the correct "scientific" view of race was clearly summarized in the Introduction to his *Politische Anthropologie:* "the biological history of the human race is the true and fundamental history of nations"; "the military and intellectual achievements of states," he continued, "can be explained in terms of the physiological features and inequality of the races which comprise them."[30] Given the degree to which Woltmann was convinced of the truth and total sufficiency of his view of race, it is not surprising that he became indignant at Schäfer and Conrad's lack of enthusiasm for his philosophy of history.

In addition to attacking the judges, Woltmann exploited his position as editor of the *Revue* to criticize Schallmayer and his treatise. Although Woltmann was able to single out one or two minor problems with Schallmayer's *Vererbung und Auslese,* the real issue was Schallmayer's outright rejection of Aryan ideologies and his reluctance to praise the work of the social anthropologists. Woltmann angrily accused Schallmayer of dismissing race theory "with empty words" and reprimanded him for "superficial arguments" used to "gloss over this difficult and little researched [race] problem." He attributed the eugenicist's stand to a lack of familiarity with the most recent literature on the subject.[31]

It would be easy to dismiss Woltmann's extreme and totally unprofessional attack upon Schallmayer and the judges as merely a case of pathological envy had it not been duplicated by several of his colleagues. Even assuming that Woltmann himself put strong pressure on Lapouge, Ammon, and others to speak out on his behalf, the social anthropologists would not have rallied to Woltmann's defense with such zeal had not more been at stake than the wounded feelings of an overly sensitive friend. Virtually the entire German Gobineau school would not have spoken out so loudly and vigorously against Schallmayer had they not perceived the outcome of the contest as a pledge of support for eugenics at the expense of their own discipline. As one social anthropologist bemoaned: "It is unfortunate that the first opportunity in Germany to support social anthropology was thwarted by the blunders in the evaluation of the entries."[32] Indeed, so strong was the need to defend the disciplinary integrity of social anthropology that Ludwig Wilser, a friend and collaborator of Woltmann, openly praised *Politische Anthropologie* as the best entry before he had even read Schallmayer's work![33]

To better understand the fears of the social anthropologists it is necessary to keep in mind that by 1904, at the time of the first critiques directed against Schallmayer and the judges, a number of eugenics-related articles and books, in particular Alfred Ploetz's influential work, *Die Tüchtigkeit unsrer Rasse* (1895) had been favorably received in various scholarly journals. Moreover, in 1904 Ploetz founded the *Archiv für Rassen- und Gesellschafts-Biologie*, (Journal for Racial and Social Biology), the organ of the incipient eugenics movement and competitor to Woltmann's *Revue*. In awarding first prize to Schallmayer, two of Germany's most eminent biologists, Haeckel and Ziegler, seemed to be supporting a movement which not only questioned the racial presuppositions of social anthropology but also threatened to become the dominant form of social Darwinism. This must have appeared all the more surprising to Woltmann and his colleagues since Haeckel was known to be sympathetic to theories upholding Aryan racial supremacy.[34]

Schallmayer responded quickly and forcefully to the criticisms and attacks of the social anthropologists. He recognized that, at least in the case of Woltmann, he was dealing with a person "whose opinion of himself was as abnormal and excessive as the volubility and lack of restraint with which he sought compensation for the injury done to his self-esteem."[35] Consequently, Schallmayer could dismiss many of Woltmann's pettier remarks as being little more than a misguided attempt to nurse his wounded pride. But Schallmayer never lost sight of the real issue: his rejection of Aryan racism. As he correctly pointed out in his *Beiträge*:

> The active apostles of modern racial ideology pay especially close attention to the way a book compares with their dogma. . . . If it ignores their views, it is worthless; if it contradicts them it is dangerous, bad, hateful and will be treated as such. In all their subjectivity . . . Lapouge, Ammon, Wilser, Woltmann and Hueppe, believe that the Jena contest could have only intended to promote science in the sense of their teachings. [They] continually reiterate that the subject matter of the prize question is the same as their race theories, although—considering the dubious scientific and even smaller practical worth of this doctrine—neither the prize donor nor any of the judges held such a view.[36]

Later on, in several articles and parts of books devoted wholly to a critique of the German Gobineau school, Schallmayer went beyond the explicit attacks of the German social anthropologists in order to highlight very important differences between his views and those of the "race enthusiasts."

From the very outset Schallmayer considered Gobineau's work to be unscientific.[37] In the second edition of *Vererbung und Auslese* (1910), however, Schallmayer directed his attack less at Gobineau than at his followers. After all, Gobineau, even if more a poet than a scientist, did have the disadvantage of writing before Darwin's views were popularized or even published. While fully recognizing the reactionary motives informing Gobineau's racial ideology,[38] Schallmayer believed that the French diplomat at least deserved the honor of being the first person to examine "cultural history from the standpoint of the hereditary worth of population *(Volkskörper)*. . . ."[39] But the modern race theorists claimed to be scientists, yet accepted the superiority of the "Nordic race" as an article of faith, as an a priori truth, in the same manner as theologians believe the teachings of the Church.[40]

Schallmayer in particular attacked the view that the "Germanic race" is the only human group capable of creating a high level of culture. This was, he thought, a classic case of unrestrained ethnocentrism. Both his first- and secondhand knowledge of Chinese civilization was enough to convince him that "the yellow race ... is, in general, scarcely inferior to the white race." The cultural values of the Chinese, he pointed out, were not the same as those of Western Europeans; indeed from the Chinese point of view, Western civilization was culturally backward.[41] Moreover, Asiatic peoples, Schallmayer continued, developed a high level of culture much earlier than the white population of Europe, and might on that basis even be viewed as superior to the Aryans. Even among Europeans, latecomers to civilization by Chinese standards, it was not "the blonde primeval race" but rather the Mediterranean peoples who first developed a flourishing civilization. Schallmayer, quoting studies by Lewis Henry Morgan and others, went so far as to suggest that "at the time of Tacitus and Caesar even the Iroquois were more culturally advanced than the Germans."[42]

Of all the presuppositions underlying the social anthropologists' theories none was more vigorously attacked by Schallmayer than the idea that mental traits could be ascribed to the various racial groups, and that these intellectual traits could in turn be deduced from physical characteristics.[43] The shape of a skull, the size of a nose, or the proportion between trunk and legs revealed nothing, he thought, about the innate mental abilities of individuals. Nor did he take seriously the German Gobineau school's discussion of racial type, racial psyche, or racial soul. Such terms were metaphysical concepts devoid of any scientific meaning.[44] Schallmayer also found ridiculous the habit of "constructing the mental characteristics" of the Nordic race using either "alleged or real intellectual traits of several outstanding personalities."[45] Even if it could be proven that Dante was blonde, it hardly followed that all Nordics were capable of composing the *Divine Comedy*. According to Schallmayer, insofar as a racial psyche existed at all, it was an infinitely complex web of all the individual mental traits of all the people belonging to the race[46]—hardly something readily accessible to the present-day researcher.

Schallmayer was consoled by the knowledge that the racial nonsense of the Gobineau school was not taken seriously by many professional groups, especially by mainline German academic anthropologists.[47] Yet this knowledge in no way lessened his fears that the aims and methodology of eugenics might be either falsely or intentionally equated with social anthropology—that race hygiene and racism, so to speak, would become linked in the public eye. A mistaken linkage of the two would serve to discredit the young discipline Schallmayer spent so much time promoting; an intentional linkage would "guide the eugenics movement in a direction that leads nowhere or nowhere good."[48]

A large part of the confusion concerning the goals of eugenics, Schallmayer thought, could be traced to the double
meaning of the term *Rasse* (race). On the one hand Rasse de-
noted "the sum of hereditary traits of any individual, usually in
the sense of hereditary fitness." On the other hand Rasse was
used to denote "a large group of individuals who, owing to their
common descent, possessed common hereditary traits which
separated them from other groups of the same species."[49]
Whereas the second meaning of race included all individuals
possessing a set of more or less common physical characteristics,
without taking into account differences in the hereditary fitness
of individuals, the first meaning focused on the variations in
hereditary fitness of individuals comprising *any* given population,
including so-called racial groups.[50] For Schallmayer, eugenics or
race hygiene was dedicated to improving the hereditary fitness
of all populations, be they composed primarily of one anthropological race or many; all human groups irrespective of
their racial, that is, anthropological, composition were equally
susceptible to degeneration and equally open to biological
improvement.

Although the two totally different ways in which Schallmayer
and the social anthropologists used the word race should have
precluded any attempt to synthesize the two disciplines,[51] the
propagandists for "racial policy" did hint that their goals could
be achieved by eugenic methods. According to the Aryan enthusiasts, the inherent worth or fitness of an individual or population depended upon the percentage of its "Nordic element";
differences between races were infinitely more important than
differences between individuals of the same race.[52] Couched in
eugenic terminology a "policy of racial supremacy" could be
carried out by encouraging only the Nordic elements in the nation to have more children, rather than all those who were biologically fittest.[53]

From Schallmayer's perspective, such a "policy of racial supremacy" was not only of dubious scientific worth but would
"lead to political and moral anarchy."[54] The racism of Woltmann,

Lapouge, Ammon, and others had already lowered Germany's prestige and popularity among foreigners.[55] Racism linked to race hygiene, however, would be even more devastating because it would ruin both the national and international respectability of eugenics. In numerous publications Schallmayer bemoaned the publicity given to the "German and Aryan enthusiasts," always comparing their endeavors unfavorably to the "true search for knowledge and wisdom" underlying the work of important eugenicists like Frances Galton.[56]

In order to minimize the confusion concerning the goals of eugenics, Schallmayer himself always employed the word *Rassehygiene* rather than *Rassenhygiene,* and continually sought to convince other eugenicists to do so. Although by 1905 the term Rassenhygiene had already been adopted by most would-be eugenicists (largely owing to the influence of Ploetz's first treatise and the *Archiv*), Schallmayer remained staunchly opposed to the plural form of the word Rasse because it excluded what for him was the most important meaning of race—race as denoting the sum total of the hereditary traits of an individual or a population.[57] He hoped that Galton's less ambiguous "national eugenics" could serve as an appropriate substitute for both terms and favored its popularization in Germany.[58] Unfortunately, however, *Eugenik* never made much headway in Germany, in part because of the reluctance of many to use an English word when an acceptable German term already existed, but also because some Aryan-minded eugenicists clearly valued the implicit double meaning of Rassenhygiene.[59] Although he waged a good battle, Schallmayer ultimately failed to persuade most of his colleagues to abandon the word; from its inception in the first decade of the twentieth century to its frightful end during the last years of World War II, the German eugenics movement was always known as the *rassenhygienische Bewegung* (race hygiene movement).

Throughout his career Schallmayer fought hard to see to it that the Aryan enthusiasts and their ideologies did not gain a foothold in the incipient eugenics movement—that race hygiene did not become racist.[60] He did not, however, meet with total success. Though the Wilhelmine and Weimar eugenics movement was not totally free of the influence of the Aryan mystique, it did not direct its program toward the propagation of a Nordic elite. Race hygiene under the swastika witnessed the complete synthesis of the two disciplines.

BIOLOGICAL EFFICIENCY AND SOCIAL POLICY

Schallmayer also came into conflict with a second group: the academic social scientists.[61] Here too professional prestige and disciplinary integrity played a significant role in the several critiques directed at both Schallmayer and eugenics. But unlike the intellectually bankrupt attacks of the social anthropologists, those of the social scientists contained wholly defensible and legitimate arguments concerning Sozialpolitik. Schallmayer and German eugenicists in general sought to make biological efficiency an important goal, if not *the* goal of social policy. The discussion of social policy and its enactment, however, was traditionally in the hands of academic sociologists and social theorists—men who, rightly or wrongly, viewed race hygiene's attempts to modify and transform social policy with suspicion or even hostility.

We have already discussed Wilhelmine Germany's obsession with what contemporaries called "the social question." Although Schallmayer's 1891 book touched indirectly upon the relationship between biological efficiency, the social question, and social policy, it was Alfred Ploetz who, in the twelve or so years spanning the publication of Schallmayer's two treatises, actually defined and fleshed out the so-called race hygiene-social policy problem. Like Schallmayer, Ploetz was interested in social and economic questions and trained as a physician before turning his attention exclusively to eugenics.[62] In 1892, while practicing medicine in the United States, he first expressed his sentiments concerning the problem in a short article published in an American socialist paper. Subsequent articles such as "Racial Fitness and Socialism" (1894), and "The Relationship Between the Principles of Social Policy and Race Hygiene" (1902), as well as Ploetz's important eugenic treatise *Die Tüchtigkeit unsrer Rasse und der Schutz der Schwachen. Ein Versuch über Rassenhygiene und ihr Verhältnis zu den humanen Idealen, besonders zum Sozialismus* (The Fitness of Our Race and the Protection of the Weak: A Discussion Concerning Race Hygiene and Its Relationship To Humanitarian Ideals, Especially to Socialism) (1895), served to convey a more detailed analysis of the issue.[63]

The major thrust of Ploetz's argument recalls Darwin's personal dilemma in the *Descent of Man:* how can human beings reconcile the inevitable conflict between the humanitarian ideals and practices of the noblest part of our nature, with the interest of the race, whose biological efficiency is impaired by those very ideals and practices. Translated into concrete economic and political terms, Ploetz viewed the problem as follows: should the state, indeed could the state, continue to expand the social net and regulate various aspects of economic life in order to lessen the hardships of the weak and economically underprivileged, at the risk of undermining the overall biological fitness of its citizens? Would not social legislation providing for health, accident, and old-age insurance invariably lead to an increase in the number of unfit, perhaps at the expense of the fittest members of society? For Ploetz, the conflict between humanitarian instincts and biological imperatives was simple; the solution, however, was less so.[64]

Ploetz's initial answer to the dilemma, as spelled out in his book, involved a form of germ-plasm selection. This germ-plasm selection, however, would not be indirect—the result of eugenic practices whereby only the fit were encouraged to reproduce—but rather direct: all married couples would be asked to select only the most superior of their germ cells for fertilization.[65] Once the laws of heredity were more exactly understood, couples could exploit this knowledge with an eye toward preventing the transmission of so-called inferior variations. As Ploetz himself pointed out, "the more we can prevent the production of inferior variations, the less we need the struggle for existence to eliminate them."[66] If couples could ensure that their offspring were their genetic superiors, the capitalist system as a form of selection would be superfluous; social legislation or even socialism could be introduced without fear of any long-term biological damage. In such a manner, Ploetz maintained, the goals of humanity could be reconciled with the interest of the race.

Ploetz's desire to master the laws of heredity as a first step in the "control of variability" reveals the same managerial-technocratic logic that underlay Schallmayer's eugenic strategy. Initially, however, Ploetz did not propose any of the more controversial eugenic measures, but instead wished to "push selection back" to the pre-fertilization stage with his plan for germ-cell selection.[67] This plan was, of course, totally unfeasible. Although he did not abandon all discussion of it, Ploetz was forced, at least temporarily, to rely on other means to achieve his end. But his adoption of some of the more traditional goals and programs articulated by Schallmayer and others did not dampen his interest in the relationship between social policy and biological fitness; he merely turned his attention to the way existing social policy either aided, harmed, or ignored the goals of eugenics.[68]

For years Ploetz wrote articles that touched on the relationship between the social sciences and race hygiene. In 1910, however, he decided to walk into the lion's den. On October 22, Ploetz presented a paper entitled "The Concepts of Race and Society and Several Problems Relating to Them" at the First Conference of German Sociologists in Frankfurt.[69] Most of the dons of German academic sociology and economics were present. After a lengthy series of definitions of terms like race, race hygiene, society, and social biology, Ploetz paused a moment to point out the ethical significance of race hygiene: Properly understood, race hygiene provided nothing less than "the final . . . normative imperative for all human action."[70] The social scientists were then treated to a discussion of the relationship between race and society which, Ploetz's description of its "symbiotic" nature notwithstanding, implied that society, and hence social policy, existed to serve the interest of the race.

Although one delegate was willing to defend Ploetz,[71] the reaction of most of the other social scientists was, if not overtly hostile, certainly far more critical of his outlook. The views of Werner Sombart and Max Weber were typical of those of many of the participants. Sombart, as chairman of the conference, had little opportunity to express his own opinions in the debate, but his sentiments on the subject of the relationship between the social sciences and eugenics were well known from an article entitled "Ideals of Social Policy."[72] Published at least in part as a reaction to Ploetz's *Die Tüchtigkeit unsrer Rasse,* Sombart's essay touched on a number of significant issues also raised in Ploetz's 1910 speech. Perhaps the most important issue was whether social policy should serve eugenic goals.[73] According to Sombart, social policy was synonymous with economic policy, and it sought only to preserve and promote a particular economic system.[74] Believing himself to have been successful in freeing social policy from the ethical concerns of older economists, Sombart was not about to bind it to another ethical ideal like race hygiene. Moreover he also remained unconvinced of the absolute priority of "the good of the species" over other ideals.[75] Indeed, for Sombart social policy and race hygiene had little to do with each other—an assessment which Schallmayer would later call into question.

Sombart also rejected the eugenicists' claim that societies behave according to natural law—an idea further developed by Max Weber at the 1910 conference. In what was the most sophisticated critique of Ploetz's views, Weber began his discussion by attacking several of the eugenicist's presuppositions. For example, Weber neither accepted Ploetz's premise that biological fitness was a prerequisite for civilization nor supported his conclusion that degeneration posed an imminent threat to society.[76] In addition, he also lashed out at the ambiguous term Rasse, a term that for Weber was totally incapable of explaining a single important sociological phenomenon.[77]

Weber reserved his most perceptive criticism for last. Deliv-

ered more in the manner of a warning than a reproach, Weber
reminded Ploetz of the dangers of making excessive claims for
the biological perspective of social events at the heart of race
hygiene:

> I should like to question the idea that, just because some processes
> which concern biology—the processes of selection—are undoubtedly
> affected by social institutions . . . it therefore makes sense to appro-
> priate any object or problem in that area for a science which has yet
> to be constructed for the first time for this very purpose. . . . We
> have seen how it has been believed that the whole world, including
> for instance, art and everything else, could be explained in purely
> economic terms. We see how modern geographers treat all cultural
> phenomena from a geographical point of view. . . . My view is that
> the individual sciences lose their point when each fails to perform
> that specific task which it, and it alone can perform; and I should like
> to express the hope that this fate may not befall the biological ap-
> proach to social phenomena.[78]

What Weber demanded of Ploetz and the other eugenicists were
empirically-based case studies demonstrating the importance of
biological factors for "concrete social phenomena." Until such
time as race hygiene was in a position to furnish "exact evidence" to support its claims (which Weber did not doubt might
someday come to pass), the new discipline should refrain from
exaggerating the usefulness of the biological approach for the
social sciences.[79]

Years before the conference, the Krupp competition provided
other social scientists with a perfect opportunity to attack the so-
called biological perspective on social phenomena. Although at
least one or two went so far as to dismiss the very possibility of
the social sciences learning anything from Darwinian biology,[80]
most of the social scientists who bothered to enter the contest
chose rather to condemn the extreme and one-sided positions
adopted by Schallmayer and the other prizewinners.

The psychologist A. Vierkandt and the sociologist Ferdinand
Tönnies were two representatives of the social sciences who
went to great lengths to attack Schallmayer's *Vererbung und Aus-*

lese directly. In an article bearing the caustic title "An Invasion of the Humanities by the Natural Sciences?" Vierkandt criticized Schallmayer's attempt to create an allegedly new scientific picture of social reality by using an extremely shaky intellectual construction, Weismann's theory of heredity, as the foundation.[81] Yet even if Weismann's theories should turn out to be correct, Vierkandt maintained, Schallmayer's totally uncritical manner of transferring the concept of selection to human culture would seriously detract from the scholarly pretensions of his book: Indeed, for Vierkandt, Schallmayer's entire discussion of social phenomena suffered from a "lack of a firm and adequate sociological foundation."[82] An examination of such difficult concepts as self-preservation, social altruism, compassion, prudery, intellect, and moral characteristics in general, was the "task of psychology and sociology," and should not be subjected to crude biological analysis. In Vierkandt's opinion, Schallmayer's entire investigation of the subject of instincts demonstrated "how a little vulgar psychology, . . . the natural ornament for scientists not professionally trained in psychology, suffices for the solution of the task."[83] Vierkandt undoubtedly viewed Schallmayer's response to the Krupp contest as an unwelcome intrusion into his discipline.

Tönnies prefaced his protracted attack on Schallmayer with a critique of the aims and pretensions of the contest. From Tönnies' perspective, it was ludicrous to attempt to ascertain the alleged meaning of the new biology for all aspects of political and social life as long as the principles of evolutionary theory remained themselves hotly disputed among biologists.[84] Indeed, the crude either/or wording of the contest question with respect to the inheritance of acquired traits led Tönnies to believe that the Preisausschreiben had less to do with the interest of science than with defending the political status quo. In short, the whole purpose of the contest was to prove that Darwin's theory was "politically correct."[85]

One might well ask, as Schallmayer did, why a person who held such a cynical view of the contest would himself bother to submit an entry. In his *Beiträge*, Schallmayer at least suggested that personal dissatisfaction with the outcome of the contest (Tönnies did not receive a prize) might have had something to do with the sociologist's sharp criticism of it. To be sure, Tönnies' attempt to hide the fact that he himself was a contestant at least calls into question the intellectual integrity of his attack upon Schallmayer.[86] But unlike Woltmann's critique, Tönnies response was not occasioned primarily by wounded pride. Both the length and depth of his arguments as well as his serious attempt to familiarize himself with the basic tenets of Galton's eugenics,[87] suggests that something more substantial than a deflated ego was at stake.

Like Vierkandt, Tönnies began his critique by accusing Schallmayer of crude selectionism in his discussion of social phenomena—a selectionism based, as he viewed it, on Schallmayer's uncritical adoption of Albert Schaeffle's analogy between the organism and the state.[88] He then turned his attention to a critical examination of the presuppositions and desirability of Schallmayer's eugenic proposals, the main target of his verbal assault.

Despite his alleged concern for the "generative interest," Tönnies viewed Schallmayer's eugenic measures, especially the refusal to grant marriage licenses to those hopelessly unfit or temporarily infected with venereal disese, as both utopian and harmful.[89] Laws designed to prevent dysgenic marriages or ensure that a syphlitic male did not infect his spouse would not, and could not, prevent extramarital sex and illegitimate children. The way to effectively eliminate the unfortunate hereditary consequences of venereal disease was not to legislate against the marriage of infected males, but rather to reduce prostitution. But the eventual elimination of prostitution involved elevating the social and economic status of women, particularly working-class women, and achieving social stability—conditions not to be brought about by eugenic laws but rather by an energetic social policy.[90]

Even more than "negative eugenics," Schallmayer's plan to encourage the so-called talented groups of society to increase their ranks deeply troubled Tönnies. Who in fact were the most talented? Tönnies attacked Schallmayer for his unproven assumption that the upper classes were necessarily fitter than other social classes. This view, Tönnies argued, was nothing more that a revised and somewhat watered down version of Ammon's doctrine of social selection, whereby class differences were linked to alleged differences in hereditary fitness.[91] But even if it could be proven that the upper classes were intellectually better, did that automatically mean that they were morally or physically superior?[92] To clarify his point Tönnies offered the example of shortsightedness, which occurs more frequently among the highly educated.[93] Should talented individuals be encouraged to reproduce even if they are myopic, Tönnies asked? Indeed the real question remained: what traits should be selected? How could social policy serve to promote the biological fitness of the nation when no agreement was possible on what constituted fitness? For Tönnies, these and similar questions rendered Schallmayer's eugenics both impractical and undesirable as a means of boosting national efficiency.

Schallmayer responded speedily and forcefully to Vierkandt and Tönnies, accusing them of disciplinary tunnel vision and deliberate misrepresentation of his views. His rejoinders to the two social scientists, however, were not nearly as significant as his attempt to defend the biological view of social policy against the attacks, charges, and innuendos leveled by German social scientists in their debates with Ploetz, a task he accomplished in his *Beiträge*. Indeed the very title of his book, *Contributions to a National Biology*, was designed to call into question the traditional idea that the economic perspective was the only correct one in dealing with social and political issues. Heretofore the economic imperative had dominated the social sciences, and social policy was more or less synonymous with economic policy. But to Schallmayer economic imperatives were definitely not enough to ensure the stability of the nation, and economics could not alone solve all of Germay's problems. "The biological-hereditary wealth of the nation," he maintained, "was certainly no less valuable for the well-being and political position of the state than its material assets. . . ."[94] The social sciences must be placed on a firm biological foundation, and the dominant economic outlook prevalent among social scientists must be replaced by a biological outlook.

In tune with the scientism of the age, Schallmayer used the opening chapter of his *Beiträge* to extol the virtues, importance, and power of natural science. Science not only promoted the material progress and technological advances necessary for Western hegemony[95] but also provided significant theoretical and epistemological insights into the nature of the universe, the origins of human beings, and the nature of the human condition. The so-called *Geisteswissenschaften* (humanities), according to Schallmayer, could boast of no significant progress in the last hundred years, in part because of the subordinate position of science, and especially biology, in the educational curriculum—a deplorable situation for which he held the church and the classically trained humanists largely responsible.[96] This being the case, it was hardly surprising that German social scientists lacked the critical biological insight necessary to analyze social problems.

This lack of input from biology, when combined with vested interests, prevented the "humanist sociologists," as Schallmayer labeled them, from adopting a "sociobiological" perspective, or even admitting that the social sciences, as they were presently practiced, were simply not making progress or solving any important problems. It was hard to deny, contended Schallmayer, that more criminals now walked the streets, that family law showed no sign of development, and that Germany's economic system, at least from the standpoint of preserving and stabilizing society, had little to be proud of. In addition, race hatred and doctrines of racial superiority were on the rise, threatening to divide individual countries and cause friction between nations. This, coupled with the ever-growing class hatred between rich and poor, suggested that something was wrong with the traditional social science perspective on social issues.[97] Social policy had not, even by its own definition, solved the social question.

For Schallmayer, the social scientists' desire to increase the economic productivity of the nation without taking its biological basis into account represented a serious shortcoming of current social theory. This viewpoint was expressed most vividly in an attack upon Sombart entitled "The Sociological Importance of the Progeny of the Talented and the Inheritance of Intelligence." After lashing out at Sombart for his desire to protect his discipline from outside interests (i.e., eugenicists),[98] Schallmayer opened fire on Sombart's theoretical presuppositions. He accused Sombart and the social scientists of assuming that national wealth alone generates culture and science, while totally neglecting the "physiological basis" or hereditary foundation of all knowledge and society.[99] Biologically ignorant social theorists, Schallmayer maintained, either viewed this hereditary foundation as an unchanging entity, or in a crude Lamarckian fashion, as something directly affected by external conditions, including improved economic conditions.

What Sombart and others failed to realize, however, was that all social development, including an increase in economic productivity, presupposed an ever-higher level of biological fitness and hereditary talent. Consequently, it was both foolhardy and dangerous to promote an economic system or social policy which might in the long run undermine the very level of biological efficiency necessary to maintain a high level of economic productivity.[100] Create a policy that favors the intellectually, morally, or physically inferior half of the population, and Germany's economic vitality was bound to decrease; develop instead a program that encourages the "fitter" groups in society to outreproduce the less fit and the Reich would prosper both economically and biologically.

But Schallmayer's criticisms of Sombart and the social scientists were not limited to their ignorance of the alleged biological basis of economic efficiency. Although he shared with them an emphasis on economic efficiency and the rational management of society to achieve their common goal of preserving and strengthening of the body politic,[101] Schallmayer's opinions differed in two very important respects. Whereas for the social scientists economic efficiency was synonymous with national efficiency, for Schallmayer other variables less immediately related to economic productivity, such as population growth, were also critical for the long-range welfare of the nation. Moreover, whereas the social scientists believed that all impediments to national efficiency could be eliminated by social and economic measures, Schallmayer held that many of the obstacles to a strong state, such as criminality, homosexuality, suicide, and mental illness, were essentially biological in nature[102] and could only be adequately removed by embarking on a eugenics program.

Arguing from his assumption that both the means and goals of politics presupposed a high level of hereditary fitness, Schallmayer stressed the need for social policy to become eugenic policy. For Schallmayer, a well-informed eugenic policy presupposed biologically-trained social scientists and government officials willing and able to examine all social, political, and economic institutions from the standpoint of their effectiveness in improving the overall hereditary fitness of the nation. The changes that would thereby come about were essentially the same eugenic measures to ensure that Germany maintain its position in the struggle for survival among nations envisaged by Schallmayer in *Vererbung und Auslese*. But, most important, eugenic policy meant that biological efficiency must become the immediate goal of social policy. Only then could the common final goal of both Schallmayer and the social scientists—national efficiency—be fully realized.

EUGENICS VERSUS HYGIENE?

In contrast to the social anthropologists and academic social scientists who distanced themselves from race hygiene, several of Germany's public hygienists were among the most active members of the incipient eugenics movement. In fact one hygienist, the distinguished bacteriologist Max von Gruber (1853–1927), went on to become chairman of the German Society for Race Hygiene in 1910. At the outset, however, many public hygienists felt professionally threatened by the so-called new hygiene. The publication of both Ploetz's *Die Tüchtigkeit unsrer Rasse* and Schallmayer's *Vererbung und Auslese,* but above all the German translation of John Haycraft's inflammatory book, *Darwinism and Race Progress,*[103] triggered a critical and defensive reaction on the part of hygienists, who viewed eugenics and its Darwinian assumptions as fundamentally at odds with the basic tenets of their discipline.

Underlying the eugenics-public hygiene controversy lay two seemingly opposed intellectual and disciplinary perspectives on the nature of social progress and national welfare.[104] The first, the biological-Darwinian, emphasized the importance of a continuous struggle for survival under harsh conditions as a necessary prerequisite for social and cultural evolution. According to the "Darwinian" interpretation, unless the number of "unfit"— the physically, intellectually, morally, and perhaps economically weak—could be reduced, or at least held in the same proportion to the overall population, biological and social decay was inevitable.

Opposed to the "selectionist" view of progress stood a large portion of the medical profession, but above all, the tradition of public hygiene. The expressed goal of the empirical/experimental science of hygiene[105] was to protect individuals from harmful external or environmental conditions which adversely affect health. Since health care was not only an individual but also a national concern, public hygiene played an important political role.[106] Although hygienists had long been conscious of their critical role in safeguarding the nation's health and welfare, only in the 1880s, largely as a result of Koch's discoveries and the subsequent rise of bacteriology, did hygienic practitioners really possess the necessary theoretical and scientific knowledge to adequately fulfill their duty as custodians of the nation's health.[107] In spite of their eventual realization of the limitations of germ theory for solving public health issues, German public hygienists remained preoccupied with the external variables at work in disease, for example, climate, nutrition, sanitation, and living conditions. They were naturally inclined to believe that improved hygienic conditions and further medical discoveries would continue to upgrade the health and vitality of the nation.

Advocates of the two conflicting traditions clashed over the role of hygiene in the so-called degeneration problem. Eugenicists and supporters of the Darwinian perspective shocked and outraged the small community of German hygienists with their assertion that public hygiene was in large measure responsible for the progressive biological degeneration of Western society. Several prestigious medical and health-care journals such as the *Münchener Medizinische Wochenschrift,* the *Vierteljahrsschrift für Gesundheitspflege,* and the *Zentralblatt für allgemeine Gesundheitspflege,* carried articles attacking the seemingly preposterous claims of men like Ploetz and Schallmayer. Some public hygienists publicly denied the existence of an ominous "degeneration problem."[108] Others, insofar as they accepted the reality of biological degeneration at all, tended to blame Entartung not on modern hygienic practices but on unfavorable environmental conditions related to poverty. As one concerned adherent of this position put it, "the degeneration question is essentially a problem of nutrition."[109]

Probably sparked in part by the publication of *Vererbung und Auslese,*[110] three prominent German hygienists employed empirical data in an attempt to settle the "degeneration problem" once and for all. Using newly available statistics on birth and death rates, infant mortality, and army recruitment, Max von Gruber, Walter Kruse, and Friedrich Prinzing sought to discredit the selectionist assumptions of the eugenicists by demonstrating a lack of any positive correlation either between high infant mortality and low child mortality,[111] or between high infant and child mortality and military fitness. They also reiterated the importance of hygiene in bolstering national health.

According to the hygienists' interpretation of the Darwinian position, a high infant and child mortality rate should increase the fitness of the adult population. Those who passed the initial selection period (from birth to age five), so the theory ran, should be less likely to die young, succumb to disease, or if male, be rejected for military service. Yet statistics, at least as the hygienists evaluated them, undercut this so-called selectionist premise. All three men presented evidence which directly contradicted the Darwinist position that high infant and child mortality resulted in increased military fitness. In fact, just the opposite was the case—high infant mortality went hand-in-hand with poor military fitness.[112] Moreover, as Gruber and Prinzing pointed out, high infant mortality did not favorably affect the future health of a population: it neither resulted in a lower child or adult mortality rate, nor reduced the percentage of adult cases of tuberculosis.[113] Indeed in Greenland, where the harsh struggle for survival should have produced individuals perfectly suited to their environment, childhood death and adult diseases were more common than among Western peoples. Although more than a quarter of all Greenland Eskimo infants died before the age of one, the mortality rate of adult Eskimos was three to four times the rate of Danes of the same age. How could Darwinists explain such unfortunate medical facts? Did "Eskimos still have too much hygiene?" Gruber questioned sarcastically.[114] Obiously, since infant mortality did not serve to improve the race, the Darwinists had no right to call into question the long-range biological implication of hygienic and medical practices aimed at lowering the number of infant and early childhood deaths.[115]

In addition to challenging the selectionist argument that high infant mortality benefited the race, the hygienists, in good Lamarckian fashion, stressed the importance of improved hygienic measures, better living conditions and, above all, the control of infectious diseases in promoting biological fitness. Kruse argued that the sharp reduction in the number of deaths resulting from infectious diseases over the past twenty years suggested an increase, not a decrease, in biological strength and vitality.[116] Moreover, contrary to the claims of the Darwinists, the hygienists asserted that harmful environmental conditions, especially contagious diseases, kept biological efficiency at a lower level than necessary. How many fatal illnesses, contended Gruber, resulted not from any deficiency in hereditary fitness but rather from noxious agents and "infectious germs" against which all individuals stood defenseless? And how many individuals became unfit not by virtue of inferior hereditary material, but only because they were improperly fed either before or after birth?[117] Stressing the importance of nutrition as a prophylactic against degeneration, Gruber even went so far as to suggest that one could raise the average biological quality of a population without improving its hereditary substrate by simply upgrading the diet of all individuals.[118] Indeed most hygienists agreed with Gruber that, insofar as public hygiene sought to eliminate hazardous environmental conditions, it benefited not just the "weak" but all members of society. To avoid degeneration and improve the health of the nation, more hygiene, not less, was needed.[119]

The hygienists' attack on Darwinism, their unwillingness to take the issue of degeneration seriously, and their insistence that hygiene did no long-term biological damage to the race, undoubtedly deeply troubled Schallmayer. Especially disturbing, indeed insulting to Schallmayer, was the hygienists' suggestion that Darwinists were heartless enemies of public hygiene who reveled in statistics of high infant mortality.[120] Refutations of individual arguments made by the three men notwithstanding, Schallmayer's rejoinder to the hygienists focused on two main issues: first, that eugenicists were not anti-hygiene and did not envisage high infant mortality as the proper means of achieving biological efficiency; and second, that degeneration and its opposite, biological fitness, was linked to and could only be properly understood in terms of changes in the hereditary substrate of a population.

Regarding the first point, Schallmayer quickly pointed out that eugenicists were far more concerned about intellectual and moral degeneration than they were about any increase in the number of physically unfit owing to hygiene.[121] That having been said, however, he insisted that one could still believe that high infant mortality played a selective role (albeit a relatively small one) in the life-process of nations, yet refuse to applaud or even tolerate such a ruthless form of selection.

> Upon examination of the facts and arguments both for and against a selective role for child mortality, we see that it does possess some selective effect. It does not follow, however, from the social eugenic standpoint, that the reduction of this imperfect and brutal method of selection should be regretted or combatted. . . . This inefficient and relatively unproductive method of natural selection cannot only be replaced, but even overcompensated for, by a rational social management of reproduction which is neither cruel nor injurious to our concepts of human integrity.[122]

Just as "no feeling human being" could oppose therapeutic medicine for preserving the life of the unfit, so too could no humane individual reject public hygiene simply because it was sometimes counterselective. Schallmayer challenged the hygienists to give an example of even one Darwinist or eugenicist who publicly repudiated the aims of hygiene. Such an individual, Schallmayer suggested, if indeed he existed, would be in need of a psychiatrist.[123] Even the extremist John Haycraft, when properly understood, could not be said to be against hygienic measures. "The eugenicist's ideal," maintained Schallmayer, "cannot be the return to an emphasis on natural selection, but rather the replacement of culturally-hemmed natural selection through the perfection of sexual or germinal selection."[124]

Schallmayer also chastised the hygienists for their alleged misinterpretation of the degeneration problem. Particularly exasperating from Schallmayer's point of view were comments made by Gruber annd Kruse to the effect that Entartung was not limited to hereditary traits.[125] Moreover, owing to their conscious or unconscious Lamarckism, the hygienists employed the term degeneration to describe all unfavorable changes in the physical and mental composition of either an individual or a population, ignoring the important Weismannian distinction between "somatic" changes—changes that do not alter the germ-plasm and are therefore not inherited—and true heredity modifications.[126] For Schallmayer, the term Entartung could only be applied to heredity traits and referred only to a negative change in the hereditary material of an individual or group. In an attempt to clarify the issue he offered the following definition of the often poorly understood concept.

> Degeneration . . . is a generational hereditary development accompanied by a deterioration of the functional efficiency of one or more physical or mental organs, which results in future generations becoming less adapted to their living conditions. . . . National degeneration [*Volksentartung*] means a decline in the average hereditary qualities of a people such that its overall fitness with respect to the demands necessitated by the struggle for survival is diminished.[127]

"Generative degeneration," Schallmayer added, occurred not only when external conditions were too favorable but also when they were so severe that no individual's germ-plasm could withstand them without appreciable damage. For Schallmayer, this explained why the Greenland Eskimos, despite their subjection to a most rigorous selection, did not demonstrate a high degree of fitness.[128]

More significant for an understanding of the development of Schallmayer's ideas than his reply to Kruse, Prinzing, and Gruber was his reaction to Alfred Grotjahn's important work *Sociale Pathologie* (Social Pathology). Grotjahn was a leader of the turn-of-the-century movement to create a separate discipline of social hygiene independent of the then-dominant experimental-biological tradition. He was also the first hygienist to recognize publicly the legitimacy of the "race hygiene" perspective, and was instrumental during the Wilhelmine and Weimar years in drumming up support for eugenics among his professional colleagues.[129] Although Schallmayer greatly admired Grotjahn for his pioneering theoretical work in the field of social hygiene, and appreciated his dedication to the cause of eugenics, he rejected

Grotjahn's classification of eugenics as a subdiscipline of social hygiene.[130]

Schallmayer found Grotjahn's view of the relationship between race hygiene and social hygiene unacceptable for one very important reason: by and large, the two hygienes strove toward different immediate (if not final) goals and employed dissimilar means to achieve their ends. Race hygiene, according to Schallmayer, was solely concerned with the hereditary fitness of a population—the quality of its inherited germ-plasm—and had as its aim the largest possible increase of "good" hereditary traits, and the largest possible decrease, if not total elimination, of "undesirable" characteristics. This goal was to be achieved primarily by altering social policy and social institutions in such a way as to encourage the so-called fitter portion of the population to out reproduce those deemed "less fit" or "unfit." Social hygiene, however, strove merely to ensure the best possible development of already existing traits. On the whole, it achieved its goal by creating a highly favorable environment or living conditions for a given population.[131] Employing the most up-to-date biological terminology, Schallmayer explained the difference as follows: eugenics represented "genotype hygiene" whereas social hygiene was equivalent to "phenotype hygiene."[132]

Besides having different ends and means, the two hygienes served different constituents. Race hygiene benefited future generations far more than it did the present generation; social hygiene aided only those presently alive and possibly their immediate descendants.[133] This difference was closely linked, Schallmayer maintained, to the dissimilarities and conflicts between what he called *Sozialinteresse* (social interest) and *Rasseinteresse* (racial or hereditary interest). An institution or measure—military recruitment for example—could be extremely valuable for the short-term social interest, yet be quite harmful from the long-term racial or hereditary perspective. In such cases of conflict national leaders were naturally faced with a tough decision. Although in principle the Rasseinteresse should always take precedence over the Sozialinteresse, in practice the basic social needs of society must first be met before the long-term racial interest could be addressed.[134] Making an intelligent judgment when conflicts between the two arise required, Schallmayer emphasized, "an improvement and expansion of sociological and socio-biological learning." He hoped that state officials and politicians would soon acquire the requisite knowledge necessary to make such important decisions.[135]

Owing to the fundamental differences between race hygiene and social hygiene with respect to goals, methods, and beneficiaries, neither field could be legitimately considered a subspecialty of the other; each, Schallmayer asserted, was an independent discipline with its own aims and programs.[136] Yet despite their basic dissimilarities, the two hygienes' separate interests occasionally overlapped. Both eugenics and social hygiene strove to reduce or eliminate harmful external agents such as alcohol, toxic chemicals, and bacteria-producing congenital diseases which impair both the health of an individual as well as his or her germ-plasm.[137] Moreover, the practitioners of the two disciplines, at least in some respects, shared the same premises and intellectual outlook. Schallmayer certainly would have agreed with the statement of the eminent social hygienist Alfons Fischer that "prophylaxis is the physician's true domain."[138] One can safely say that social hygienists and eugenicists alike stressed the superiority of preventive medicine over therapeutics, and viewed their disciplines as prophylactic. In fact, although race hygiene was largely a reaction against the one-sided public preoccupation with the successes of the newest subspecialty of hygiene, bacteriology, the possibilities which bacteriology held out for a truly effective preventive medicine gave eugenicists like Schallmayer reason to believe that they too could eradicate disease once and for all instead of merely treating it. Despite differences in their methodology and focus of attention (hygienists concentrated on the carrier of disease, eugenicists on the bodily constitution), eugenicists and hygienists shared a common belief in and were influenced by the prevailing ideology of scientific medicine. In addition, practitioners of the two hygienes shared a common attitude about the relationship between health and society. Both sought to regulate social policy in such a way that it furthered the health of the nation, however differently they interpreted the term health. And finally, as medical professionals, eugenicists and social hygienists were both conscious of their social and political role as guardians of the nation's health and well-being—although each believed that it made the more important contribution to the cause.

Their common presuppositions concerning the political role of the medical professional, the relationship between health and society, and the importance of preventive medicine may explain why so many hygienists, once convinced that eugenics did not seek to put them out of business, became actively involved in the race hygiene movement. Certainly many hygienists must have come to the same position as Max von Gruber that race hygiene was both a prerequisite for and an extension of any long-term social hygiene program.[139] At any rate, Schallmayer himself was convinced of the necessity of both hygienes, since both—albeit in different ways and in varying degrees—promoted national efficiency.

For Schallmayer, eugenics and social hygiene were part of a larger overarching "biological policy" or "national biology"—a systematic program to upgrade the biological fitness of the nation.[140] This program can be graphically portrayed as shown in figure 1.[141] As indicated by the sketch, race hygiene together with personal and social hygiene, comprised what Schallmayer termed "qualitative population policy." As the name suggests, this part of Schallmayer's biological policy had as its aim the improvement of the biological quality of the population. One portion of qualitative population policy, namely eugenics, served the racial or hereditary interest; the other part, personal or social hygiene, benefited the immediate social interest. The other half of biological policy, quantitative population policy, sought to regulate social institutions and practices such that they promoted the largest possible increase in population. Here the emphasis was on quantity, not quality of population—with one

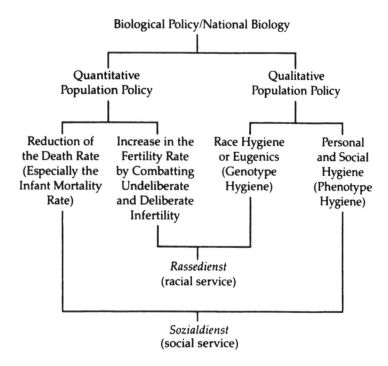

Figure 1.

part enhancing the racial hereditary interest, the other merely aiding the social interest.

Schallmayer's biological policy or national biology was a comprehensive plan to help boost national efficiency. Indeed he designed all his programmatic statements with the same goal in mind. His insistence, for example, that eugenics refrain from ideologies of Aryan supremacy was rooted in his belief that no one anthropological race had a monopoly on useful hereditary traits. The difference between the social productivity of two individuals of the same race could far exceed that of any two individuals belonging to different races. Schallmayer's demand that social policy become race hygiene policy also reveals his preoccupation with national efficiency. Only by promoting biological efficiency, Schallmayer asserted, could the eugenicists' and socal scientists' common desire for a strong and stable state be fully realized. And, finally, underlying both Schallmayer's support of public or social hygiene and his effort to convince hygienic practitioners that race hygiene was not their enemy was his firm belief that both hygienes, their fundamental differences notwithstanding, aided the cause of national efficiency.

Thus far we have examined Schallmayer's "qualitative population policy." After 1908, and especially during World War I, however, Schallmayer and the incipient eugenics movement became particularly involved with the other pillar of biological policy: "quantitative population policy." The origins of Schallmayer's interest in the population question and his formulation of a "population policy" is the subject of the next chapter.

V

POWER THROUGH POPULATION: SCHALLMAYER AND POPULATION POLICY

Statesmen and social philosophers have long appreciated the dialectics of population and power; population was viewed by ancient Greek political theorists, French mercantilists, and German cameralists as a source of national strength and wealth. By the turn of the century, the belief in the necessity of maintaining a large and vigorous population had become a mainstay of the then-popular social Darwinist outlook. For Schallmayer, a large population was a prerequisite for economic efficiency and cultural progress, both of which were absolutely imperative for any nation wishing to hold its own in the ever-present international struggle for survival.[1] Only *fruchtbare Völker* (fertile nations), he warned, could sufficiently recover from the twin scourges of war and epidemic without being overrun by others.

Yet despite his recognition of the importance of population *quantity*, Schallmayer spent the early years of his career almost exclusively preoccupied with population *quality*, that is, with eugenics in the narrow sense of the term. Given his interest in promoting a eugenic consciousness in Germany, Schallmayer's choice of emphasis hardly seems surprising. What is significant, however, is his shift of focus from quality to quantity of population beginning around 1908—a shift which by 1915 led him to view the prevention of a decline in population growth as "a matter of survival for the German nation."[2] But why did this change come about at this particular time? In order to understand the obsession of Schallmayer and other German eugenicists with the population question, as well as their efforts to formulate a concrete *Bevölkerungspolitik* (population policy), it is necessary first to draw attention to certain significant prewar demographic, social, and political changes in Germany which undoubtedly colored their intellectual perspective.

BIRTHRATE DECLINE, NEO-MALTHUSIANISM, AND PREWAR PARANOIA

Germany during the Wilhelmine era was the second most populous country in Europe. Between 1871, the year of unification, and 1910, the population of Germany increased by about twenty-four million, from forty-one to nearly sixty-five million—an increase representing a doubling time of just under seventy years.[3] Yet despite its healthy growth in population Germany, like all Western industrial countries, experienced a steady birthrate decline during the last third of the nineteenth and first third of the twentieth century. Demographers are unable to offer a precise date for the beginning of the decline in Germany's birthrate—significant regional variations make such a task impossible—but it may safely be said that by 1880 a statistically meaningful decline was underway.[4] After about two decades of a relatively slow decline, a steady and much faster drop in the number of births occurred around 1902. For example, in the twenty years between 1880 and 1902 the birthrate fell from 37.6 per thousand inhabitants to 35.1—a decline of 2.5 live births. However, between 1902 and 1914, a period of only twelve years, Germany suffered an 8.3 per thousand drop in the number of live births.[5] Because of the larger proportion of women of childbearing age, and the increase in nuptiality,[6] the marital fertility rate declined even faster than the birthrate, which proved especially disconcerting for eugenicists like Schallmayer.

Population growth continued despite the sharp drop in fertility, primarily because of the even more rapid decline in the death rate, particularly the infant mortality rate. Ignoring the very significant statistical differences between various social classes and regions of the country, improved living conditions as well as medical and public health advances did cause a lowering of Germany's notoriously high infant mortality rate—from 26.0 per thousand inhabitants in 1880 to 16.2 in 1910—with large cities such as Berlin demonstrating a particularly rapid decline.[7] Although Germans could rightly be proud of these reductions in the number of infant and early childhood deaths, the steady decline in the excess of births over deaths after 1902 still gave statisticians and eugenicists cause to expect an eventual population standstill or even population decline.[8] The continuous stream of German emigrants to North and South America coupled with the drastic reduction of the number of immigrants (mostly Polish agricultural laborers) coming into the Reich only served to worsen what for many was an alarming problem.[9]

The declining birth and fertility rates generated both interest and concern among Germany's statisticians, social theorists, and medical professionals. Although the pioneering empirical studies of statisticians like Arthur von Fircks, Marcus Rubin, and Harald Westergaard already reflect a growing awareness of the population question as early as the 1890s, the first attempts to discuss Germany's declining fertility in its larger socioeconomic context did not appear until after 1900.[10] In perhaps the most influential of all post-1900 studies, the liberal social theorist and economist Lujo Brentano proposed what became popularly known as the *Wohlstandstheorie* (prosperity theory): "Improvements in the standard of living . . . instill mobility aspirations as well as a desire for even greater material wealth, and the limitation of family size [is] . . . one way to realize these goals."[11] In short, as prosperity increases fertility decreases.

Many of Brentano's contemporaries, however, took issue with this interpretation. As an alternative, the influential government advisor and Berlin professor Julius Wolf postulated a relationship between declining fertility and what he termed *Ordnungssinn* (a sense of bringing one's affairs in order).[12] As the general level of education rises and an awareness of the desirability, if not necessity, of remaining economically solvent sets in, individuals come to view children as a possible drain on the family economy and hence seek to avoid having too many. A couple need not be well off, as the Wohlstandstheorie suggests, before it decides to limit the size of the family; in the interest of getting ahead even individuals with very modest means might seek to better themselves by having fewer children.[13]

Other concerned individuals offered still different explanations for the declining birth and fertility rates. Reinhold Seeberg, a member of the consistory of the Prussian Protestant Church, blamed the drop in fertility on a steady decline in religiosity and a rise in both egotism and naturalism.[14] Those not satisfied with monocausal explanations suggested a combination of many factors such as the rise in prostitution and venereal disease, the burgeoning growth of the cities, as well as the influence of liberal and socialist ideologies. But whatever their differences (and they were considerable), all statisticians held two things in common: (1) they were less alarmed by the actual decline in population growth than by the prospect that Germany's situation might soon begin to mirror French demographic realities, where the introduction of the two-child system actually resulted in population decline;[15] and (2) they were convinced that the drop in fertility rate was conscious and directly related to the promotion of birth control methods by supporters of Neo-Malthusianism.

The origins and growth of Neo-Malthusianism in Germany have yet to find their historian.[16] It seems quite possible, however, that the German movement, if one can indeed call it such, received its impetus and theoretical direction from the English Malthusian League.[17] Founded in 1877, and later counting many distinguished social reformers and feminists among its members, the English Malthusian League sought to update Malthus's solution to the so-called population problem without challenging the basic presuppositions of the controversial early nineteenth-century economist. Accepting Malthus's position that poverty resulted from the extreme fecundity on the part of the working-class poor, the modern or "neo"-Malthusians, who backed the League, rejected his prescription of late marriages and self-restraint as both "unnatural" and "unhealthy," and substituted instead the idea of family planning through contraceptives.[18] Underlying their support of modern birth control practices lay the classical liberal assumption that the greater the reduction in the number of laborers, the higher the wages of the working class. Birth control, by raising both wages and the overall standard of living, necessarily improved national health and even had, as many argued, a positive eugenic effect on the race.[19]

Like its English counterpart, German Neo-Malthusianism was closely linked to both the feminist movement and the changing social position of women—indeed the two were totally interconnected. Despite entrenched legal discrimination against German women and their need to battle an illiberal political system, middle- and upper-middle-class women did enjoy new opportunities in work and education at the turn of the century not available a generation earlier.[20] For the great majority of women, work was certainly more a question of financial necessity than a means to promote personal growth and independence, but the large influx of female labor into the work force and the impressive increase in the number of female white-collar workers, especially after 1900,[21] could not help but chip away at the traditional stereotype of *Kirche, Küche,* and *Kinder* (church, kitchen, and children) as the only acceptable female roles. Such gradual changes in attitude on the part of both female workers and society as a whole undoubtedly altered the social position and social consciousness of women.

More important from the standpoint of the feminist movement, by 1900 German women had gained access to that bastion of male supremacy, the university. Whereas before 1890 there were few, if any, women attending German universities, in 1905 some eighty women were enrolled full-time, and by 1914 the number of female students pursuing academic degrees had increased to 4,126.[22] Many women entering the university prepared for a medical career; the great majority, however, trained to become elementary and secondary schoolteachers—a trend that precipitated important reforms in German girls' education.[23]

It was the educated middle-class woman, as Schallmayer continuously bemoaned, who fueled the fire of Germany's growing women's movement. Although dating back to 1865, the bourgeois women's movement gained more organizational coherence and adopted a more progressive stand with the establishment in 1894 of the Bund Deutscher Frauenvereine (Federation of German Women's Associations).[24] While hardly qualifying as a monolithic unidirectional social force, the women's movement basically remained true to the unpopular ideas of political liberalism in late Wilhelmine Germany,[25] and concentrated on two main concerns: female suffrage and sexual reform.

Sexual reform became the movement's key issue during its short-lived radical period in the mid-1900s.[26] For those German women who went beyond the modest demands of more conservative leaders like Helene Lange, sexual reform encompassed a whole series of issues collectively known as the "new morality." Reduced to its bare essentials, the new morality attempted to deal with the practical problems affecting unwed mothers while simultaneously attacking the taboo placed on extramarital sex.[27] It would be wrong, however, to dismiss it as merely a means to advance the cause of sexual liberation. As its adherents saw it, the new morality defended the right of women to become self-conscious, free individuals able to lead productive and intellectually meaningful lives.[28] As such, it naturally rejected all attempts to reduce the sphere of women's activities to the traditional three Ks (Kirche, Küche, and Kinder). In order to achieve its aims of female emancipation, many prominent new morality advocates such as the feminist Helene Stöcker turned to birth control and Neo-Malthusianism. Disgusted with the conventional view of marriage as merely a means to "secure the continuity of the race and the preservation of the state," Stöcker saw in Neo-Malthusianism "one of the most effective means of solving the woman questions and indeed the social question in its entirety."[29] Stöcker and her like-minded feminist supporters in the *Bund für Mutterschutz und Sexualreform* (League for the Protection of Motherhood and Sexual Reform) continued to press for "individualistic" aims such as sex education in the schools, birth control, and repeal of the antiabortion statute, while at the same time devoting attention to the practical problems facing unwed mothers.[30]

The decline in fertility, which was allegedly caused in part by this anti-baby and anti-motherhood propaganda of the feminists and Neo-Malthusians, became all the more disturbing to Schallmayer and others in view of the deterioration in the international political climate after 1900. Direct challenges to European hegemony and the growing belief in the possibility of war made Germany's falling birthrate appear far more ominous than it would have seemed just a decade or two earlier.

German eugenics, like similar movements elsewhere in Europe, must at least in part be understood in the context of the gradual decline of European political and cultural world leadership. Degeneration was reported to be a phenomenon specific to Western industrialized *Kulturvöker,* and self-styled degeneration theorists in all European nations with an active eugenics movement turned their attention toward saving the European cultural elite—the educated middle classes—from a sort of biological extinction. More often than not eugenicists stressed the internal menace: the rising tide of allegedly genetically inferior and unproductive individuals (often associated with the unskilled working-class poor). But there were also, at least in the eugenicists' minds, external foreign dangers which threatened to eclipse the preeminence of Europe in global affairs: the "yellow peril" and the rising Slavic threat.[31]

After 1900 many thoughtful Europeans developed, as historian Geoffrey Barraclough has aptly pointed out, "an almost neurotic awareness of the precariousness of their position in the face of an expansive Asia."[32] Contributing to this awareness was the rise of Japan to world power status following its victory over Russia in 1905. For the first time in modern history a European power fell victim to an Asiatic state. Exacerbating the resulting fear was the rise of violent anti-European sentiment in China during the Boxer Rebellion (1899–1900), which, together with rapid population growth and a long cultural tradition, raised the specter of a revitalized China even more powerful than Japan.[33] For eugenicists like Schallmayer who were acutely aware of European demographic trends, Asia's burgeoning population growth, together with its potential military superiority, spelled both political and biological danger for the entire white race.[34]

With the breakdown of Bismarck's diplomatic policies after his dismissal as chancellor in 1890, and with the subsequent formation of new European alliances, fear of the "Russian bear" vied with, if not surpassed, the "yellow peril" in the minds of most war-conscious Germans. After all, it was not China or Japan but rather Russia, with its population of roughly 105 million and its army of over a million men, which bordered on the Reich and was allied with Germany's potential enemies, England and France. The fear of encirclement, which arose from the realignment of the major powers, was magnified by the perceived danger of a disproportionate increase in the number of Russians and other Slavs, which in the words of Schallmayer, would cause "for us firstly, an unfavorable change in the military balance of power *vis-à-vis* the east European states, and secondly, a correspondingly large emigration from the same which would result in the increasing Slavization of Germany."[35]

The ostensible Slavic threat and fear of "encirclement," the "yellow peril," and the growing militarization of Germany combined to turn the population problem into a national crisis. The same statisticians who, on one page, calmly and objectively reported Germany's falling fertility rate, often ended that account with a grave warning that Neo-Malthusianism, and the resulting decline in population growth, would inevitably be advantageous to either the Asians, the Russians, or both.[36] Hence it was hardly an accident that by 1908, in the context of this conjunction of circumstance—birthrate decline, Neo-Malthusianism, and pre-war paranoia—Schallmayer, like other German eugenicists, began to focus his attention on the population problem and devote his energies toward remedying it.

SCHALLMAYER'S ANALYSIS
OF THE POPULATION PROBLEM

Once convinced of both the reality and danger of Germany's declining birthrate, Schallmayer took pains to try to analyze this unfortunate trend by examining its contributing factors. Four categories or factors quickly came to mind as being particularly significant: bachelorhood and spinsterhood, late marriages, involuntary reduction in fertility, and most important, conscious or voluntary reduction in fertility.[37] As Schallmayer proceeded with his analysis, it became increasingly clear that besides stunting Germany's population growth, the above-mentioned factors also had a distinctly dysgenic effect on the nation's level of hereditary fitness. Fertility decline inevitably meant a drop in biological efficiency.

Regarding the first factor, Schallmayer employed statistics and case studies to demonstrate the impact of bachelorhood and spinsterhood on both the quantity and quality of population. In 1910 nearly one-third of the male population between twenty and sixty remained single permanently, he reported. The percentage of single women was even worse; in 1900, 46.5 percent of women between the ages of fifteen and fifty—almost one-half on all adult females—never married.[38] For Schallmayer the net loss in population growth resulting from such a large number of single people was a serious problem in its own right. If, however, one also took into account the fact that a disproportionately large percentage of those remaining single were from the educated middle and upper-middle classes, the situation appeared even more critical.

Late marriages, especially prevalent among the "higher social classes," only compounded the problem. According to statistics available to Schallmayer, between 37 and 38 percent of German women waited until after age twenty-five to marry; indeed, only 9 to 10 percent married before their twentieth birthday.[39] To make matters worse, only modern Western industrialized countries experienced such gloomy nuptial realities. In Russia, as Schallmayer was quick to point out, over half of the brides were under twenty—a fact that accounted for the nation's high fertility rate[40] because a correlation existed between the age at which a woman married and the number of children she was likely to bear. Schallmayer, quoting Galton's figures, argued that the fertility of women who marry at twenty-nine compared with that of women who marry at twenty stood in a relationship of five to eight, an entirely unsatisfactory state of affairs when one considered the type of women who tended to marry later in life.[41] And since the trend toward late marriages had always been even more extreme among men, especially educated career-oriented men, Germany's biological strength and vitality were doubly threatened.[42]

Not unrelated to late male marriages was the third category of involuntary reduction in fertility. Disregarding the relatively minor impact of chronic alcoholism on fertility, venereal disease was interpreted by Schallmayer to be the single most important cause of unintentional infertility. Reaching epidemic proportions, especially in the large cities, venereal disease accounted for a high percentage of miscarriages and stillbirths and, at least according to one of Schallmayer's sources, 40 to 50 percent of all childless marriages.[43] Moreover, like bachelorhood and late marriages, the spread of venereal disease not only resulted in the loss of thousands, perhaps millions of healthy and productive adults, but also adversely affected population quality. Since educated middle-class and upper-class men were more often than not forced to marry late, they were faced with the alternative of either repressing their "sex drive" for an unnaturally long period of time or resorting to a prostitute—the latter frequently leading to gonorrhea.[44] Few, according to Schallmayer, could be satisfied with the first option. What this meant, in short, was that these infected but eugenically superior males were likely to subject

their future spouses to possible lifelong sterility, robbing themselves, their wives, and their country of talented progeny.

But whatever the negative impact of bachelorhood and spinsterhood, late marriages, and venereal disease on fertility, it was
completely overshadowed by the kind of conscious family planning made possible by birth control practices. At one time high
nuptiality virtually assured high fertility, but now, as demographic trends in France painfully demonstrated, an increase in
the number of marriages went hand in hand with birthrate decline. Superficially, at least, "modern, relatively safe and not ex-
cessively uncomfortable male and female contraceptives,"
Schallmayer insisted, were to blame.[45] Yet the availability of birth
control devices did not, Schallmayer knew, really explain why
couples tended to have fewer children. Rising material expecta-
tions, greater educational career opportunities, and above all, an
increase in individualism were, in a more meaningful sense, at
the root of the population problem. For Schallmayer, all three,
but especially the last, nurtured Neo-Malthusianism in Germany.

A bitter opponent of Neo-Malthusianism all his life, Schallmayer began lashing out against its propaganda campaign during the fear-ridden prewar years. Neo-Malthusian supporters, he
affirmed, simply failed to realize that they were leading the nation toward disaster; they were not the true heirs of the famed
English economist. Malthus, unlike the Neo-Malthusians, at least
understood the necessity of having a large population, and never
advocated artificial contraception. The Neo-Malthusians,
however, not only stressed the usefulness of contraceptive devices but also attempted to "convince the public that a large
number of children was not, as formerly believed, a blessing, but
rather, something wrong and shameful, a moral blemish, both
for the rich and poor."[46] Moreover, they either ignorantly or
maliciously preached that their birth control practices actually
benefited the race.

Nothing irritated Schallmayer more than the Neo-Malthusians' erroneous claim that family planning improved the biological substrate of the general population. Annoyed and concerned
that such a view went unchallenged, Schallmayer seized the op-

portunity to set the record straight when, in 1908, he was given the chance to review the widely read and influential book, *Race Improvement, Malthusianism, and Neo-Malthusianism*. The author of the treatise, the Dutch Neo-Malthusian advocate Johannes Rutgers, had become one of the most prominent leaders of the international birth control movement. He seems to have been especially popular among certain German feminists—so much so in fact that Marie Stritt, then president of the Federation of German Women's Associations, wrote the introduction to the German translation of Rutgers's work.[47] Like many other supporters of Neo-Malthusianism, especially those in England, Rutgers honestly believed that his birth control crusade promoted the eugenic cause, and was both surprised and disappointed to find out that Germany's leading eugenicist did not agree with him.[48]

Of Rutgers's numerous claims disputed by Schallmayer in his review article, the two most important and hotly contested were the Dutch physician's assertion that a declining fertility rate did not spell race suicide or national downfall, and his contention that birth control had an advantageous selective effect on any given population.

In his attack on the first point, Schallmayer accused the "crack-brained Marxist" of gross historical ignorance; only a narrow-minded Social Democrat could maintain that those concerned about the population problem were nothing more than imperialists worried about having enough cannon fodder in case of war.[49] Schallmayer, hardly a warmonger, was decidedly more concerned about the eclipse of cultural hegemony allegedly resulting from a falling birthrate. Remember, argued Schallmayer, that "the French have declined not only as a military power but also in cultural importance in the wake of the spread of Neo-Malthusianism."[50] But even more ominous than a decline in France's position as cultural leader of Europe was the threat facing all European nations as a result of the "yellow peril."

If the flabby views and comfortable habits for which the Neo-Malthusians and feminists make propaganda become dominant among the white civilized nations, the white race will not only not expand over the Earth, but will doubtlessly . . . sooner or later either be militarily defeated by the tough and rapidly growing portion of the yellow race and then be gradually replaced by its reproductively superior competition until it [the white race] disappears, or, if hostilities are avoided by all sides, the peaceful immigration of the fecund Asiatics . . . will lead to exactly the same result.[51]

Although admittedly couched in racialist terms, Schallmayer's suggestion was not that the Asians were necessarily biologically or culturally inferior to whites. They were simply different and, owing to large and ever-increasing numbers, seemed to pose a threat to the values and culture he held dear.

Schallmayer found Rutgers's second claim—that birth control had a positive selective effect on the race—equally fallacious. The Neo-Malthusian slogan "improvement of racial quality through limitations on quantity" was theoretically bankrupt, for in practice, and that was what counted, birth control had an unmistakable dysgenic effect. The "degenerates," as Schallmayer pointed out, were not the ones employing birth control.[52] Since it was mostly educated, middle-class women who with the aid of contraceptives practiced a kind of maternal selection, Neo-Malthusianism promoted not racial improvement but rather racial decay.[53] Moreover, those women who practiced birth control did not do so for noble reasons (e.g., to save themselves and their country the pain of a possible defective child), but merely because the infant was personally or financially inconvenient. Such "individualistic discretion," Schallmayer complained, was as compatible with the "demands of a successful generative ethics as water with fire."[54] In sum, far from being a racial blessing, Neo-Malthusianism was decidedly "antieugenic."

Birth control and family planning were also advocated by German feminists—often, to be sure, as part of their overall acceptance of the basic tenets of Neo-Malthusianism. Yet just as Schallmayer declined to blame Neo-Malthusianism directly for the declining fertility rate, so too was he reluctant to attribute Germany's falling birthrate to the success of the women's movement; both were said to be merely manifestations of an ostensibly prevalent obsessive individualism.[55] Directly related to the individualism championed by the feminists was their position on the issue of motherhood. Despite the great diversity within the women's movement, complained Schallmayer, almost all feminists "consider only a very modest dose of motherhood worthy of women."[56] German feminists, especially liberal "new morality" advocates like Helene Stöcker, placed great emphasis on the right of women, if primarily middle-class women, to lead intellectually rewarding lives inside and outside the family. That intellectual growth and career development were often hampered, if not totally curtailed, by the physical and mental drudgery of repeated pregnancies and child care was only too clear to the feminists. Their somewhat less than enthusiastic support of motherhood reflected their liberal and libertine convictions.

Needless to say, the generally low esteem in which at least some prominent German feminists held motherhood directly contradicted and threatened the basic tenets of Schallmayer's eugenic thought. Although he did not explicitly say it, Schallmayer undoubtedly agreed with his Dutch colleague, sociologist Sebald Steinmetz, that "if it actually becomes customary for all talented women to choose an independent career . . . only those too dumb, too weak, or those who have too little stamina will devote themselves entirely to motherhood."[57] In Schallmayer's opinion it was patently absurd that the most talented and biologically desirable women went off to work while the less intelligent and biologically undesirable stayed home and had children. Apologizing in advance for his remark, Schallmayer offered the following comparison: "Whereas in horse-breeding the best animals are employed for reproduction and the remainder for work, in modern human society just the opposite is the case."[58] For Schallmayer, men could always hold jobs presently filled by women; "by far the most important task that a hereditarily fit woman could accomplish was reproduction."[59]

If, as Schallmayer certainly believed, fecundity was of paramount importance for national efficiency, a cult of motherhood had to be created whereby childbearing would be made to seem desirable. It was necessary to elevate motherhood to a high-status, dignified occupation—one with a sense of moral and national significance. Such a revised, eugenically informed cult of motherhood must find its way into the elementary and secondary schools. There girls would be taught at an early age the racial and national importance of reproducing according to their degree of biological fitness.[60] Eventually, Schallmayer hoped, such education might produce a new generation of high-minded and ethically motivated women who would be willing to place their personal and individualistic interests below those of the race and nation. He even contemplated a time when the entire women's movement would itself embrace the ideal of motherhood—a time when former feminists would become *Bundesgenossinnen* (powerful and indispensable comrades) working together for a common cause: biological efficiency.[61]

SCHALLMAYER, WORLD WAR I, AND POPULATION POLICY

The coming of war, and especially the realization after 1915 that the fighting was likely to continue far longer than originally anticipated, only intensified both Schallmayer's and Germany's concern over the population question. Evidence of the growing anxiety over declining population growth and the factors contributing to it can be seen in the formation of several organizations during the war years which were either directly or indirectly preoccupied with redressing the population problem. One of the most important of these societies, and one to which Schallmayer belonged, was the Deutsche Gesellschaft für Bevölkerungspolitik (German Society for Population Policy), founded in 1915. The society, which counted among its over one hundred members numerous high-level civil servants, physicians, economists, statisticians, and religious leaders, set itself the following tasks: first, to encourage Germans to have children; and second, to alter existing "material conditions" so that large families became financially feasible.[62] In addition to these major goals, the society stressed "the national importance of the occupation of housewife" and the education of girls for a career as mother and housewife. It also declared an all-out war on the spread of venereal disease.[63] Other organizations dedicated to promoting population growth, like the Bund zur Erhaltung und Mehrung der deutschen Volkskraft (League for the Preservation and Increase of German National Strength) with membership in 1915 of one thousand, expressed aims which were similar to those of both the German Society for Population Policy and the German Society for Race Hygiene.[64]

Perhaps most indicative of the degree of national concern over the population question was the German government's active participation, beginning around 1915, in discussions, meetings, and organizations designed to tackle the problem. Prior to the outbreak of hostilities, the government appears to have been completely indifferent to the warnings and pleas of German eugenicists; the numerous calls for eugenics-related reforms, including proposals designed to promote population growth, went unheeded. Nor is there much evidence to suggest that the government was even seriously paying attention to eugenic propaganda before the war.[65] By 1915 however, the connection between the military needs of the Reich and a large and healthy population was too obvious to be ignored, and government officials began to take a more active interest in putting an end to Germany's falling growth rate. In that same year Chancellor Bethmann-Hollweg sent a representative to the first meeting of the Society for Population Policy. Less than two years later, the government was officially represented at an important conference held at the Royal Agricultural College in Berlin. There, representatives of nineteen societies concerned with the problem of insufficient population met to discuss what could be done to remedy the situation.[66]

From Schallmayer's perspective, the government's growing eugenic awareness was the only positive development to emerge from the outbreak of hostilities. Even had he not viewed modern warfare as dysgenic and counterselective, Schallmayer's pacifist tendencies and cosmopolitan outlook precluded any enthusiasm for the war, in contrast to more nationalistic eugenicists like Gruber and Fritz Lenz (1887–1976). Although he never openly condemned the war, Schallmayer frequently lamented the continued fighting, and especially took pains to inform his readers of the anticipated biological cost of the hostilities. As was mentioned earlier, the war merely aggravated his pre-1914 anxiety about the population question; Schallmayer did not, by and large, alter his stand on Neo-Malthusianism, birth control, or the women's movement. But whereas before the war Schallmayer was more frightened of "the fecund Asiatics" than the Russians, after 1914 it was the latter that, in his opinion, posed the most serious and immediate national danger. "A decision concerning the existence or nonexistence of an independent Germany in the face of the Russian threat will hardly be more than a few decades forthcoming," Schallmayer warned not long after the fighting began.[67] Russia was in a much better position to overcome its expected enormous loss of population than was Germany, and would hence continue to menace not only the Reich and its allies but indeed all Europe.[68]

But even without the Russian threat, the biological consequences of the war for Germany were anything but trivial. For Schallmayer it was painfully clear that both the short-term and the long-term impact of the present crisis on the biological efficiency of the Reich would far exceed that of the Franco-Prussian war. Not the mere 45,000 casualties of 1870–71, but hundreds of thousands, perhaps millions of able-bodied, "above-average" men (and their potential progeny) would be lost to the nation following the current war—a loss that, over time, was bound to alter the hereditary substrate of the Reich. Also, as a result of the extraordinary number of projected deaths and permanently incapacitating injuries on the front, Germany would inevitably be left with a formidable *Frauenüberschuß* (excess of women), a very serious problem in Schallmayer's mind.[69] The anticipated numerical imbalance between the two sexes meant that the birthrate was apt to sink even more dramatically than during the prewar years, since so many women would be unable to find husbands. Many women would engage in extramarital sex, Schallmayer reasoned, but because of the high infant mortality rate among illegitimate children, such promiscuity could never compensate for the rapidly falling number of legitimate births. Moreover, the availability of a surplus of women might make men more reluctant to take on the responsibility of marriage and family, since they could undoubtedly find someone willing to satisfy their needs without a marriage certificate. This, Schallmayer feared, would serve only to increase the already alarming number of women infected with venereal diseases acquired during the war, and hence cause a further reduction in the national birthrate.[70] Indeed, so serious was the biological impact of the war that a decline in population, not merely slower population growth, was a distinct possibility.[71] Both quantitatively and qualitatively, Germany's population problem was now more acute than ever before.

Anxiety in the certain decline in the level of Germany's biological fitness as a result of the war prompted Schallmayer and other eugenicists to devise a Bevökerungspolitik—a series of reform plans and programs—to help offset the anticipated quantitative and qualitative population loss. In a chapter entitled "Volksvermehrungspolitik" (Policy for Population Increase) in his thoroughly revised third edition of *Vererbung und Auslese*, Schallmayer brought together many of his own proposals with several recommended by Gruber, Lenz, and others.[72] In addition to the numerous suggestions and plans to remedy the population problem articulated by Schallmayer and others prior to 1914, such as early marriages, the fight against venereal disease, and the campaign to lower infant mortality, the chapter included several novel proposals, of which only five of the most important will be discussed here.

Although it would be difficult to try to rank-order the various proposals cataloged in *Vererbung und Auslese* according to their anticipated effectiveness in replenishing the Reich's stock of human resources, Schallmayer was certainly very favorably impressed by a suggestion first initiated by Gruber to reform Germany's inheritance laws. According to Gruber's plan, a family estate could be inherited in full only if the deceased father had left at least four children. In the event that fewer were reared, a portion of the inheritance would be turned over to relatives—presumably those with children.[73] Schallmayer, conscious of the sad state of the national treasury, offered a revised plan whereby a portion of the estate not inherited would be turned over to the Reich.[74] Either way, Schallmayer maintained, such an inheritance reform would not only boost population growth but would also encourage a higher fertility rate among the propertied classes—those classes that on the whole were eugenically more desirable.

Another population policy measure adopted by Schallmayer was the creation of free or very inexpensive homes or *Heimstätten* (homesteads) for returning soldiers and, if enough resources became available, for other "suitable" people.[75] The idea behind this plan was to make large families financially feasible for returning disabled soldiers who because they were unable to work could not afford to marry or have children, even though they were physically capable of providing the Reich with progeny. Schallmayer's scheme was undoubtedly influenced by the far more völkisch plans of Gruber and Lenz. Lenz from the outset had made the *bäuerliches Leben* (rural life) the center of his eugenic program for the biological renewal of Germany. He recommended the creation of rural homesteads and colonies to be built on land taken from Russia in the east.[76] These homesteads would be given free to eugenically desirable couples on the condition that they have at least five children. These estates could be inherited only if the parents lived up to their part of the bargain. In cases where the couple were unable or unwilling to have the requisite number of children, a fixed rent would be established.[77] Although Schallmayer did not necessarily share Lenz's nationalist and imperialist war aims (i.e., to use former Russian territory as a site for a homestead policy designed to stem the tide of the "Slavic flood"), he did believe that the establishment of such colonies would be desirable for national efficiency.[78] Echoing

Lenz, he argued that it was only fair that couples with large families be given free housing and land since such parents "provide a greater service for the race and state than they would paying rent." Presumably, if they had to pay rent, they could not afford to have as many children.[79] Like the proposal to reform the inheritance laws, the creation of such homes or homesteads, Schallmayer maintained, would enhance the quality as well as the quantity of the German population.

In addition to the two measures just discussed, Schallmayer advanced three further proposals designed to remedy the population problem: (1) the development of a state "progeny insurance" program whereby all individuals earning enough money to pay taxes would be required to give a portion of their income to a state fund that would be used to help couples with large families pay the expenses of rearing their children; (2) a wage reform for civil servants such that the more children an individual had, the higher his salary, and (3) a reform of the voting laws such that all men over twenty-five would receive as many votes as he had dependent family members (i.e., wife, daughters, and sons not yet old enough to vote).[80] These three proposals, like the two measures described earlier, were articulated and discussed by a number of eugenicists and eugenics-minded reformers in addition to Schallmayer. In fact, these and similar measures became the *Leitsätze* (guiding principles) for the German Society for Race Hygiene in its fight against the declining birth rate.[81]

None of the above-mentioned proposals and programs was ever officially adopted by the government or written into law. They are, however, worth mentioning in detail because they demonstrate the degree to which Schallmayer as well as other prominent German eugenicists viewed a large and "healthy" population as the prerequisite for national efficiency, or indeed national survival. All eugenicists knew that population, especially a hereditarily healthy population, meant power. Of course, not all population policy measures advanced the cause of biological fitness. Some proposals, like the reform of voting rights, did not discriminate between so-called genetically inferior and superior fathers. Yet on the whole the assortment of plans and programs adopted by Schallmayer and discussed at the meetings of the German Society for Race Hygiene followed Lenz's maxim: "the largest degree of fitness of the greatest possible number."[82] Only by simultaneously encouraging population quantity and quality could Germany hope to escape the biological and political damage brought on by the war.

When the war ended in humiliating defeat for Germany on November 11, 1918, Schallmayer had less than eleven months left to live. Although he never made public his feelings concerning the outcome of the war, there is every reason to believe that, like most educated middle-class Germans, Schallmayer was both shocked and horrified at the indignity of the Treaty of Versailles, and not a little dismayed at what the future would hold for his war-weary fatherland. However, unlike several of his eugenicist colleagues who were pushed to the right by events surrounding the revolutionary and counterrevolutionary activity in Bavaria, and particularly in Munich between 1918 and 1919, Schallmayer changed neither his intellectual position nor his politics during the first year of the Ebert government.[83] Whereas for Lenz, Social Democracy was equivalent to the Bolshevism he both hated and feared, Schallmayer accepted the new order, though not too enthusiastically. He had, after all, always believed that capitalism was a dysgenic and inefficient economic system, and the new leaders of the Weimar government did not appear to favor a *Pöbelherrschaft* (mob rule). From beginning to end, Schallmayer upheld the ideal of a meritocracy—a Leistungsgesellschaft—with a Leistungsaristokratie forming the ruling class.[84] Whatever reservations he might have had about the Republic, Schallmayer was certain that his dream of a meritocratic society had at least as much, if not a better chance, of becoming a reality under the new order. Had he lived longer, he would have been painfully disappointed.

EPILOGUE: SCHALLMAYER, ARYAN RACISM, AND THE LOGIC OF GERMAN EUGENICS

On October 4, 1919, after many years of suffering from various heart ailments and a severe case of asthma, the sixty-two-year-old Schallmayer succumbed to a heart attack. At the time of his death, in addition to his major prizewinning work and two other lesser known treatises, the intellectual father of the German eugenics movement had published forty-two articles in some of Germany's most prestigious medical, social science, and eugenics journals. His unquestionable intellectual importance for the development of German race hygiene was not unrecognized by his fellow eugenicists. For Hermann Siemens, Schallmayer was a "pioneer for race hygiene in our fatherland";[1] Gruber called the Bavarian physician "the first German to fully comprehend the enormous import . . . of Darwin's . . . laws for the human species."[2] But it was Lenz, one of the most influential race hygienists during the Weimar and Nazi years, who offered the most complementary assessment: "no one has accomplished more [than Schallmayer]"; his *Vererbung und Auslese* remains the "classical masterpiece of German race hygiene" and its author "enjoys a world-wide reputation, especially in England and America."[3]

Despite their sincere respect for Schallmayer's contribution to the field, Gruber's and Lenz's appraisals were not completely frank. Although during the last years of the Wilhelmine period both men stressed the same general concerns as Schallmayer, one important issue separated them from the man they eulogized: the issue of Aryan supremacy. Schallmayer, of course, was adamantly opposed to the racist connotation of Rassenhygiene—so much so that he never employed the word himself. In his view, race hygiene neither presupposed the absolute superiority of any so-called anthropological race, nor did it strive to improve one "race" at the expense of another. Though Schallmayer was certainly not without personal prejudices concerning the relative value of the three major races, he made no attempt to rank-order the various "racial groups" within the white race, for he believed the differences to be meaningless, or at best superficial. Even in cases where he felt that something approaching "racial superiority" could be discerned (e.g., in examining differences between whites and blacks), racial differences always remained less significant than class differences among individuals of the same race.[4] However, owing to their sympathies for *Germanentum*, others like Gruber, Lenz, and Ploetz found the double connotation of Rassenhygiene both expedient and desirable, and did nothing to prevent Aryan ideologues from joining the movement.[5]

Not only did Ploetz and his like-minded colleagues tolerate Aryan enthusiasts, they even catered to them. In 1911, only six years after the creation of Germany's first professional eugenics society, Ploetz, Lenz, and a physician named Arthur Wollny founded a secret "Nordic Ring" within the German Society for Race Hygiene. Its aim was the improvement of the Nordic race. As an unpublished pamphlet entitled *Unser Weg* (Our Way) points out, Ploetz and his sympathizers in the Nordic Ring harbored plans for a "Nordic-Germanic race hygiene"—if only as a part of a much broader eugenics program—which would direct its attention to saving the allegedly culturally superior Nordic elements in Western civilization.[6] In addition, these same men helped establish other similar, though not secret, völkisch organizations, including the little-known and totally insignificant Munich-based Bogenklub (1912) and the Deutsche Widar-Bund (1919). The latter, created in the aftermath of Germany's humiliating defeat, was not only pro-Aryan but also anti-Semitic and extremely nationalistic.[7] Although unsuccessful, these völkisch organizations and subgroups, to which Schallmayer never belonged, were in large measure responsible for the growing tendency, especially after the war, to equate race hygiene with the aims of "racial anthropology."

Ploetz and Lenz's defense of the ambiguous term *Rassenhygiene* and their decision to keep the movement open to Aryan enthusiasts were decidedly self-serving. Their own sympathies for the Nordic race notwithstanding, they were willing to do anything to attract the greatest number of qualified individuals to the movement, and that included capitalizing on the inroads made by the social anthropologists and other völkisch thinkers. Yet it cannot be stressed enough that even those eugenicists who sympathized with Aryan ideologies were concerned first and foremost with promoting the purely meritocratic, class-based eugenics so visible in Schallmayer's writings. Ploetz, one of the founders of the society, did not equate "fitness" with any particular race, but rather tended to view it, as did Schallmayer, in terms of social and cultural productivity. Lenz echoed Ploetz's understanding of the term: "Productivity and success in social life serve as a measure of the worth of individuals and families."[8] The *Archiv für Rassen- und Gesellschafts-Biologie,* Germany's major eugenics journal founded in 1904, was all but free of any völkisch articles, even after 1933. The concerns articulated in the *Archiv* were the same as those of Schallmayer and other nonracist German eugenicists. Prior to the Nazi period most of the entries were concerned with so-called degenerative phenomena, the dysgenic effects of certain social institutions, the social and economic costs of protecting the weak, and the "population problem." Moreover, throughout the Wilhelmine and Weimar periods *Aufnordung* (Nordification) was never a preoccupation of any German eugenicist; nor was a Nordic or Germanic heritage a prerequisite for joining the society. Physical, ethical, intellectual, and economic "fitness," however, were criteria for membership, at least during the society's early days.[9]

The overriding importance of the meritocratic tendency throughout the pre-Nazi period can perhaps best be seen in a statement made by Gruber on the occasion of Schallmayer's death:

> Even if one were convinced that Nordic blood is something particularly precious [*ein ganz besonders kostbarer Saft*], one must agree with Schallmayer that it would be a futile beginning, and more than that, a dangerous mistake leading to new discord, to want to one-sidedly select out the Nordic race from the racial mixture represented by Germans as well as other European peoples. . . . The desired goal of race hygiene can only be the unprejudiced promotion of the reproduction of the fittest and most valuable, and the limitation of reproduction of the least valuable and unfit—in a word *individual selection* within separate peoples (i.e., historically developed linguistic and cultural groups), without allowing external characteristics of anthropological races to be the sole deciding factor.[10]

Despite the preoccupation of some prominent German eugenicists with the "Aryan cause," it would be wrong to speak of two separate subdivisions within race hygiene, one meritocratic, and one racist or völkisch. Even during the politically troubled Weimar years, when differences over the race question were at their height, there was no official split in the society.[11] Instead the entire movement prior to the Nazi takeover was meritocratic, with some eugenicists and some chapters of the society also entertaining the possibility of a more limited "Aryan race hygiene." Nor should one think that Schallmayer's nonracist race hygiene was atypical, even among those in the vanguard of the movement. During the Wilhelmine period it was shared by one of Germany's most prominent eugenicists, Alfred Grotjahn. Throughout the Weimar Republic, Schallmayer's antiracist stance was continued by prominent eugenicists such as Hermann Muckermann (1877–1962), director of the Eugenics Department of the Kaiser-Wilhelm-Institut für Anthropologie, menschliche Erblehre und Eugenik in Berlin, and Artur Ostermann (1876–?), senior health official in the Prussian Ministry of Welfare and editor of the popular Berlin-based eugenics journal, *Zeitschrift für Volksaufartung und Erbkunde*, founded in 1926.

Yet even if one wishes to stress the differences between individuals on the compatibility of Aryanism and the goals of race hygiene, the technocratic logic underlying German eugenics remains the same for all adherents. The degree to which the logic so clearly articulated by Schallmayer had permeated the thinking of other race hygienists, indeed the society as a whole, can be seen in a statement made by the geneticist and eugenicist Erwin Baur, chairman of the Berlin chapter, together with two others, in a form letter written during World War I. In what was a clear attempt to elicit contributions for the creation of eugenics research institute, Baur appealed to the patriotic sentiment and good economic sense of those Germans in a financial position to help their cause:

> Will there be enough German men who recognize the hour of fate and who are ready to make sacrifices for the health of the national body [*Volkskörper*]? Huge sums are offered for private welfare; but would it not be more expedient to prevent invalidism and [hereditary] inferiority by means of an energetic race hygiene? In the future we will have to economize our resources in all areas. *Race hygiene is the prototype of a prudent rational management of human life.*[12]

The language of efficiency and the logic of managerial control over population to reduce future social costs is unmistakable.

The openness with which this logic was advanced was further strengthened during the late Weimar years. The harsh realities of the 1929 Great Depression and the constant demand to dismantle the welfare state revealed, in the crassest terms, the relationship between race hygiene and other forms of rationalization, and the cost-benefit analysis underlying both:

> Civilization has eliminated natural selection. Public welfare and social assistance contribute, as an undesired side effect of a necessary duty, to the preservation and further reproduction of hereditarily

diseased individuals. A crushing and ever-growing burden of useless individuals unworthy of life are maintained and taken care of in institutions at the expense of the healthy—of whom a hundred thousand are today without their own place to live and millions of whom starve from lack of work. Does not today's predicament cry out strongly enough for a "planned economy," that is, eugenics, in health policy?[13]

Appearing in the Preface to the Berlin-based race hygiene journal *Eugenik*,[14] a publication with a circulation of over five thousand and an editorial board which included both racist society members (Lenz) and nonracists (Muckermann), this statement is testimony not only to the astute marketing strategy of its author but also to the real nature of eugenics. Race hygienists judged individuals according to their social productivity; those deemed to be a national liability—people who, in the words of Muckermann, "cannot be brought back to work and life,"[15]—must be institutionalized as cheaply as possible. Their tainted germplasm, however, should under no circumstances be passed on to future generations. Only *Vorsorge* (foresight) in the form of eugenics could prevent generations of increased *Fürsorge* (welfare).

The necessity for concerned bureaucrats and eugenicists to find alternatives to pouring ever-increasing sums of money into institutions for the insane, the feeble-minded, and the criminal resulted in an extensive lobbying campaign for a sterilization law. Although by 1930 many eugenicists desired mandatory sterilization for the "unfit," such a position was still seen as politically inopportune. In Prussia, a law was drafted in 1932 which sought to halt the tide of the unfit by permitting the "voluntary" sterilization of certain classes of genetically defective individuals. It was supported by both racist and nonracist eugenicists and made no mention of sterilization on racial grounds.[16] Unfortunately for its advocates the political turmoil following the deposition of the Prussian government by the Reich in July 1932 ensured that the draft never found its way into law under the Republic. This did not, however, stop the requests by officials of several of Germany's state governments and members of the medical establishment for such a law. The Deutsche Ärztever-einsbund (German Physicians' Association League) specifically demanded a sterilization law not merely to prevent a deteriora-tion of Germany's *Erbgut* (genetic wealth) but also to "relieve the public treasuries."[17]

Envious of American, and to a much lesser extent, Swiss and Danish achievements in the field, many German race hygiene enthusiasts undoubtedly wondered if their own efforts to create a coherent and effective eugenics policy (including, of course, a sterilization law) would ever be realized; political and economic conditions under the Weimar government had always seemed to preclude any large-scale legislative breakthrough.[18] It was for these reasons that at least some eugenicists, such as Lenz, turned to the National Socialists as the only party capable of translating eugenic rhetoric into action. The NSDAP, as Lenz pointed out in an article written even before Hitler came to power, was the first political party to make race hygiene "a central demand of their program."[19] Lenz quoted several passages from Hitler's *Mein Kampf* to show that the latter, although possessing only a high school education, understood the necessity of embarking on a program of both negative and positive eugenics. While it is im-possible to know just how many German eugenicists shared Lenz's general, if not unqualified,[20] enthusiasm for Hitler's plans, the Führer wasted little time once he seized power in 1933 in making sure that "whoever is not physically and mentally healthy and deserving" refrain from "perpetuating his misfor-tune in the body of his children."[21]

In July 1933, a little less than six months after Hitler took office, the Nazi government wrote into law the Gesetz zur Ver-hütung erbkranken Nachwuchses (Law for the Prevention of Genetically Diseased Offspring).[22] Based on the 1932 Prussian proposal initiated by Muckermann and others, the Gesetz al-lowed for the mandatory sterilization of those individuals who, in the opinion of an *Erbgesundheitsgericht* (genetic health court), were afflicted with any of a number of "genetically determined" ailments including "feeble-mindedness, schizophrenia, manic depressive insanity, genetic epilepsy, Huntington's chorea, genetic blindness, deafness, or even 'serious alcoholism.'"[23] Although it is not known for certain who composed the law, the Gesetz was hammered out in the Sachverständigenbeirat für Bevölkerungs- unds Rassenpolitik (Expert Committee for Population and Racial Policy), a government appointed committee comprised of the eugenicists Ploetz, Lenz, and Ernst Rüdin (1874–1952), head of the German Research Institute for Psychiatry in Munich, as well as a number of racial theorists and members of the party. Rüdin, who chaired the Sachverständigenbeirat, and two Nazi officials, Arthur Gütt and Falk Ruttke, wrote the well-publicized interpretive commentary on the law.[24]

Like the earlier unsuccessful proposal to establish a sterilization law, the Gesetz was designed to ensure that a wide variety of "unfit" (i.e., "unproductive") persons did not pass on their defective hereditary substance to future generations. In Reich Minister of the Interior Wilhelm Frick's assessment, the Gesetz was necessary to prevent an otherwise inevitable decline of "fitness and German culture."[25] Mandatory sterilization of the "unfit" was hence a racial imperative. But it was also seen, at least in part, as a "legal answer" to the medical establishment's growing criticism of the "welfare state mentality." A five million dollar investment in sterilization, it was argued, could save the Reich an estimated $385 million in welfare costs and "charity support of future generations."[26] For physicians and, above all, psychiatrists trained in the hereditarian tradition of German medicine, there could be little doubt that a sterilization law would result in a significant long-term reduction in the amount of money spent on the upkeep of the "defective." In short, to the medical managers of national efficiency, it promised to be a viable cost-effective technology.

That these medical managers were singularly unconcerned with the individual fate or feelings of the "managed" hardly needs to be stressed. Although the human cost — especially the cost to women — of the Nazi state's program to prevent "undesired births" can scarcely be evaluated by mere statistics, suf-

fice it to say that from 1934 until the beginning of the war roughly 360,000 people were sterilized — more than thirty-five times
the number reported as having occurred in the United States
between 1907 to 1930 — the overwhelming majority against the
will of the individual involved.[27] Since the physicians and judges
manning the approximately 250 Genetic Health Courts employed *Lebensbewährung* (social worth), at least after 1936, as the
overriding criterion in their decision for or (rarely) against sterilization, it is hardly surprising that a large majority of the victims
were poor and/or deviant from the bourgeois norm.[28] Embracing
as it did the same logic as Schallmayer's eugenics, the Gesetz was
a measure that the Bavarian physician, had he been alive, might
well have endorsed. Since the Gesetz made absolutely no provi-
sions for sterilization on racial grounds, Schallmayer could not
have rejected it for its Aryanism.

During their twelve years in power the Nazis succeeded in
passing several other antinatal measures intended to "improve
national health." The 1935 "Law for the Protection of the Genetic
Health of the German People" required couples to undergo a
medical examination prior to marriage, and forbade marriage
between people suffering from venereal disease and certain genetic disorders[29] and differed little from measures demanded by
many Wilhelmine and Weimar eugenicists. The 1933 law against
"habitual criminals" was somewhat more draconian than any
pre-Nazi proposals insofar as it called for the forced castration of
certain categories of male "sex criminals."[30] Pronatal strategies
designed to save "valuable births" included a far stricter enforce-
ment of the antiabortion law (whereby after 1943 the death
penalty could be applied in "extreme cases"), the introduction of
marriage loans and child allowances to "valuable" couples, as
well as the bestowing of the nonmonetary "Mother Cross"
award.[31] The new guardians of the germ-plasm of the Reich
were aided in their task by the creation of a centralized system of
State Health Offices; the approximately 12,000 officials working
in the various regional offices set themselves the task of creating
a national card index of the genetic worth of all Germans to

serve as data for future state population policy decisions.[32] In this the Nazi government was taking Schallmayer's long-forgotten plea for a comprehensive set of medical statistics to its logical extreme. Heredity, as Schallmayer long-ago demanded, was finally and firmly "taken into account."

For the Nazis, however, nonracist measures such as the sterilization and antiabortion laws, and more ambiguous strategies such as marriage loans and child allowances were by no means the only or even the most important steps that needed to be taken. Hitler and his confidants now had the chance to translate their Aryan ideologies and anti-Semitic rhetoric into action, and "race hygiene" was often used as a convenient label to cover all Nazi racial policies. Consistent with the Aryan worldview of the new Reich, race hygiene as practiced and preached by the eugenicists in the newly "co-ordinated" society[33] not only had to make room for the "Nordic ideal" (which people like Ploetz, Lenz, and Rüdin were only too anxious to do) but indeed set itself the goal of "improving the Nordic race." Those like Muckermann and Ostermann who were unwilling or not trusted to follow the new official line were ousted from their positions. Jewish eugenicists such as the geneticist Richard Goldschmidt were expelled from the now wholly "German" eugenics movement.[34] As a sign of the times the nonracist journal *Eugenik* was terminated. In addition, the word *Eugenik*—often associated with left-wing tendencies in the Weimar movement and tacked on to the name of the Deutsche Gesellschaft für Rassenhygiene in 1931 as a means of placating the movement's nonracists—was eliminated as part of the society's official title.[35]

Although a new blatantly Aryan (and sometimes explicitly anti-Semitic) line is clearly discernible even among professional eugenicists such as Lenz, Rüdin, and Eugen Fischer (1874–1967), anthropologist and Director of the Kaiser-Wilhelm Institut in Berlin, this did not eliminate the older concerns of race hygiene. In addition to the various nonracist laws previously mentioned, eugenics textbooks published or used in the Third Reich differed little from those written earlier by pro-Aryan race hygienists except in emphasis and in the mandatory lip-service paid to anti-Semitism. If anything, eugenics under the swastika witnessed an even larger preoccupation with population policy and the pro-creation of the fit than had been the case earlier. One has only to examine the flood of pamphlets and books devoted to increasing the birth-rate in the "fitter" classes and reducing the number of the nonproductive to demonstrate the continuity with the past.[36] Hence during the Third Reich the definition of "fitness" became broader than had previously been the case. Whereas the race hygiene movement had heretofore always harbored many secret and not-so-secret Aryan enthusiasts, yet continued by and large to favor a purely meritocratic eugenics, post-1933 race hygiene contained not only a meritocratic component, *Erbpflege* (genetic care) but also a clearly articulated racial component, *Rassenpflege* (racial care).[37] It would thus be incorrect to assume that even Nazi eugenics was obsessed solely with Aryan themes.

But the most important continuity between pre- and post-1933 eugenics is the logic. Race hygiene presupposes a relationship between population and power. Behind Schallmayer or any other eugenicist's intention to apply "human reason to human selection" lay a technocratic conception of population as a natural resource that, in the interest of national efficiency and state power, should become subject to some form of rational control. It is quite easy to see the applicability of this logic to the creation of a stronger Nazi völkisch state. To convince the "fitter" (that is, more productive) elements in the nation to increase their number and to discourage the "unfit"—in Nazi terms not only the nonproductive but also non-Aryan population—from reproducing was to lay the biological foundations for the Thousand-Year-Reich. And to embark on a "euthanasia" action which sent over 100,000 "useless eaters" (primarily mentally ill and retarded patients) to their deaths between 1939 and 1941 was logical from the standpoint of national efficiency, as morally perverse as this logic may appear.[38]

Finally, one might add, to categorize people as "valuable" and "valueless," to view people as little more than variables amenable to manipulation for some "higher end," as Schallmayer and all German eugenicists did, was to embrace an outlook that led, after many twists and turns, to the slave-labor and death camps of Auschwitz. Most historians of the Nazi period and the Holocaust have come to recognize that despite the archaic, mystical, or otherwise irrational discourse of Nazi völkisch thought, Nazi racial practices ranging from marriage and sterilization laws to genocide presupposed highly scientific, technological, and bureaucratic methods for their execution.[39] By labeling individuals "defective" or "valueless" eugenicists in effect created a "surplus population" that could then be controlled, physically and mentally abused (as were individuals forced to undergo sterilization), and even exterminated. Of course there were also institutional links between eugenics and the "final solution" (such as the eugenicists' use of organs extracted from concentration camp victims for their "scientific research").[40] Although it would be wrong to hold Schallmayer personally responsible for the Holocaust in any way, the logic underlying his eugenics was one amenable to a project which, had he lived to witness it, would probably have caused him to question his life's work.

NOTES

INTRODUCTION

1. Emphasis mine. The German text is: "Der Staatsmann, dessen Sinn nicht blos auf Augenblickserfolge gerichtet, und dessen Gesichtskreis durch das Licht der Descendenztheorie erhellt und erweitert wäre, würde erkennen, daß die Zukunft seines Volkes von der guten Verwaltung seines generativen Besitzes abhängt . . ." Schallmayer's figurative use of the term "generativen Besitzes" is impossible to translate literally. He is obviously talking about the reproductive capabilities of the individuals comprising the nation. But even if one translates *Volk* as "people" or "race," their "generativer Besitz" would still refer to their ability to reproduce. Wilhelm Schallmayer, *Vererbung und Auslese im Lebenslauf der Völker: Eine staatswissenschaftliche Studie auf Grund der neueren Biologie* (Jena: Gustav Fischer, 1903), 380–381.

2. It is a little known fact that there were eugenics movements in countries with such disparate traditions as Canada, Russia, Norway, Sweden, Italy, Argentina, Mexico, South Africa, India, China, and Japan, as well as others.

3. There is an enormous secondary literature dealing with the history of eugenics in Britain and the United States. Anyone interested in becoming acquainted with this literature can do no better than to turn to the exhaustive "Essay on Sources" in Daniel J. Kevles, *In the Name of Eugenics: Genetics and the Uses of Human Heredity* (New York: Alfred A.

Knopf, 1985). Kevles's account of the development of Anglo-American eugenics provides a very readable and useful introduction to the subject. It is also the only book to date that offers a comparative study of the British and American movements.

4. For a discussion of the differences between French and Anglo-American eugenics, see William Schneider, "Toward the Improvement of the Human Race: The History of Eugenics in France," *Journal of Modern History* 54 (1982): 268–291, and "Eugenics in France," in *New Perspectives on the History of Eugenics*, ed. Mark B. Adams (New York: Oxford University Press, forthcoming). For eugenics in Brazil, see Nancy Leys Stepan, "Eugenics in Brazil, 1917–1940," in *New Perspectives on the History of Eugenics*.

5. The German term *Rassenhygiene* (race hygiene) had a broader scope than the English word "eugenics." It included not only all attempts aimed at "improving" the hereditary quality of a population, but also measures directed toward an absolute increase in population. Despite these differences I will employ the two terms interchangeably. Even when German eugenicists limited themselves to measures which fall under the more limited term *Eugenik* (the Germanized form of the English word), they almost always employed the term Rassenhygiene.

6. Pauline M. H. Mazumdar, "The Eugenists and the Residuum: The Problem of the Urban Poor," *Bulletin of the History of Medicine* 54 (1980): 204–215; and Donald MacKenzie, "Eugenics in Britain," *Social Studies of Science* 6 (1976): 501. Similar misconceptions appear elsewhere. For example, William Schneider, a historian of the French movement, has labeled German eugenics a "story . . . unfortunately all too familiar." Schneider, "Toward the Improvement of the Human Race," 268.

7. See for example Daniel Gasman, *The Scientific Origins of National Socialism: Social Darwinism in Ernst Haeckel and the German Monist League* (New York: American Elsevier, 1971) and George L. Mosse, *The Crisis of German Ideology: Intellectual Origins of the Third Reich* (New York: Grosset and Dunlap, 1964). In addition, authors who have written histories of race theory in its wider European context have looked at Wilhelmine eugenicists to assess their contribution to the long march to the "final solution." To their surprise, they found that eugenicists did not always hold "völkisch" views. Instead of trying to find out their real concerns, scholars still focus on the contribution of race hygienists to race theory. The following are just some examples of this: Günter Altner, *Weltanschauliche Hintergründe der Rassenlehrer des Dritten Reiches* (Zurich: EVZ, 1968); Leon Poliakov, *The Aryan Myth: A History of Racist and Nationalist Ideas in Europe*, trans. E. Howard (New York: New

American Library, 1977); George L. Mosse, *Toward the Final Solution: A History of European Racism* (London: J. M. Dent and Sons, 1978); Patrik von zur Mühlen, *Rassenideologien: Geschichte und Hintergründe* (Berlin and Bad Godesberg: J. H. W. Dietz, 1977).

8. The first studies to break away from an emphasis on Aryan racism in discussing German eugenics have tended to view it solely as an intellectual outgrowth of social Darwinism. The following are typical: Hedwig Conrad-Martius, *Utopien der Menschenzüchtung: Der Sozialdarwinismus und seine Folgen* (Munich: Köse, 1955); Hans G. Zmarzlik, "Sozialdarwinismus in Deutschland als geschichtliches Problem," *Vierteljahrshefte für Zeitgeschichte* 11 (1963): 246–273; Fritz Bolle, "Darwinismus und Zeitgeist," *Zeitschrift für Religions- und Geistesgeschichte* 14 (1962): 143–178; Gunter Mann, "Rassenhygiene—Sozialdarwinismus," in *Biologismus im 19. Jahrhundert in Deutschland,* ed. Gunter Mann (Stuttgart: Ferdinand Enke, 1973), 73–93; Mann, "Biologie und der 'neue Mensch,'" in *Medizin, Naturwissenschaft, Technik und das zweite Kaiserreich,* ed. Gunter Mann and Rolf Winau (Göttingen: Vandenhoeck und Ruprecht, 1977), 172–188; Mann, "Neue Wissenschaft im Rezeptionsbereich des Darwinismus: Eugenik—Rassenhygiene," *Berichte zur Wissenschaftsgeschichte* 1 (1978): 101–111. While nobody can deny the intellectual importance of social Darwinism for eugenics, the problem with these explanations is that they give the reader the impression that social Darwinism, by itself, *caused* eugenics. Others working on the history of eugenics have portrayed it, consciously or unconsciously, as a humanitarian attempt to improve the human race that was perverted by the Nazis. See, for example, Werner Doeleke, *Alfred Ploetz (1860–1940): Sozialdarwinist und Gesellschaftsbiologe* (Med. diss., Frankfurt, 1975) (Tübingen: privately printed, 1975) and Georg Lilienthal, "Rassenhygiene im Dritten Reich. Krise und Wende," *Medizinhistorisches Journal* 14 (1979): 114–133. The issue of humanitarianism in eugenics is tricky. While I do not doubt that some eugenicists (especially Schallmayer) sincerely had the interest of their countrymen and nation at heart and saw eugenics as a means of eliminating hereditary illness, etc., this does not *explain* the appearance of the phenomenon. Lilienthal's main point, however, is to show how an allegedly neutral and objective science (German eugenics before 1933) became corrupted and misused during the Third Reich. But Lilienthal's claim that there was a *wertfrei*(neutral) eugenics is unacceptable. Insofar as all eugenicists upheld social productivity as a criterion for fitness, race hygiene was obviously value-laden, even in those cases when it was free of ideologies of Aryan supremacy.

9. Gerhard Baader, "Das 'Gesetz zur Verhütung erbkranken Nachwuchses'—Versuch einer kritischen Deutung," in *Zusammenhang. Festschrift für Marielene Putscher,* eds. Otto Baur and Otto Glandien (Cologne: Wienand, 1984), 865–875; Gerhard Baader and Ulrich Schultz,
eds., *Medizin und Nationalsozialismus: Tabuisierte Vergangenheit—Ungebrochene Tradition?* Dokumentation des Gesundheitstages Berlin 1980, I
(Berlin-West: Verlagsgesellschaft Gesundheit mbH, 1980); Gisela Bock,
*Zwangssterilisation und Nationalsozialismus. Studien zur Rassenpolitik und
Frauenpolitik,* Schriften des Zentralinstituts für sozialwissenschaftliche
Forschung der Freien Universität Berlin, Bd. 48 (Opladen: West-
deutscher Verlag, 1986); Klaus-Dieter Thomann, "Auf dem Weg in den
Faschismus: Medizin in Deutschland von der Jahrhundertwende bis
1933," in Barbara Bromberger, Hans Mausbach, and Klaus-Dieter
Thomann, *Medizin, Faschismus und Widerstand. Drei Beiträge* (Cologne:
Pahl-Rugenstein, 1985); Hans-Martin Dietl, et. al., *Eugenik. Entstehung
und gesellschaftliche Bedingtheit,* Medizin und Gesellschaft, Bd. 22 (Jena:
VEB Gustav Fischer, 1984); Hans-Peter Kröner, "Die Eugenik in Deutschland von 1891 bis 1934" (Med. diss., Münster, 1980); Jürgen Kroll, *Zur
Entstehung und Institutionalisierung einer naturwissenschaftlichen und
sozialpolitischen Bewegung: Die Entwicklung der Eugenik/Rassenhygiene bis
zum Jahre 1933* (Sozialwiss. diss., Tübingen, 1983) (Tübingen: privately
printed); Georg Lilienthal, *Der "Lebensborn e. V.": Ein Instrument nationalsozialistischer Rassenpolitik,* Forschungen zur neueren Medizin-
und Biologiegeschichte, Bd. 1 (Stuttgart and New York: Gustav Fischer,
1985); Benno Müller-Hill, *Tödliche Wissenschaft: Die Aussonderung von
Juden, Zigeunern und Geisteskranken 1933–1945* (Hamburg: Rowohlt,
1984); Paul Weindling, "Die Preußische Medizinalverwaltung und die
'Rassenhygiene.' Anmerkungen zur Gesundheitspolitik der Jahre
1905–1933," *Zeitschrift für Sozialreform* 30 (1984): 675–687; Weindling,
"Race, Blood and Politics," *The Times Higher Education Supplement,* 19
July 1985: 13; Weindling, "Soziale Hygiene: Eugenik und medizinische
Praxis—Der Fall Alfred Grotjahn," *Das Argument: Jahrbuch für kritische
Medizin* (1984): 6–20; Weindling, "Weimar Eugenics: The Kaiser
Wilhelm Institute for Anthropology, Human Heredity and Eugenics in
Social Context," *Annals of Science* 42 (1985): 303–318.

10. Schallmayer, *Über die drohende körperliche Entartung der Kulturmenschheit und die Verstaatlichung des ärztlichen Standes* (Berlin: Heuser,
1891).

11. The term *national efficiency* as used throughout this book derives
from G. R. Searle's history of the English national efficiency movement,
*The Quest for National Efficiency: A Study in British Politics and Political
Thought, 1899–1914* (Oxford: Blackwell, 1971). Britain's "national efficiency movement" began as a reaction to Britain's dismal showing during

the Boer War and the fear surrounding Britain's decline as a major power. Including members of all political parties and persuasions, the movement sought to replace what was considered to be an outworn Gladstonian (liberal) approach to governing nation life by an emphasis on scientific and state planning in the interest of making the nation more competitive. Although Germany never had a national efficiency movement per se, and the term was never used, the second industrial revolution and the growing competition between imperialist powers made the concern for the achievement of the maximum possible power with least expenditure of resources a prevalent concern among politicians and social theorists in Wilhelmine Germany.

12. Throughout this study the term *nonracist eugenicist* will be used to describe those race hygienists who rejected ideologies of Aryan supremacy. This is admittedly a very narrow definition of the word *nonracist*. Like most European intellectuals of their day, all eugenicists were racist in the sense that they believed in the natural inferiority of blacks and most other so-called nonwhite races.

1: SOCIAL, PROFESSIONAL, AND INTELLECTUAL ORIGINS

1. Ralf Dahrendorf, *Society and Democracy in Germany* (New York: Anchor, 1969), 33.

2. Walther G. Hoffmann, "The Take-Off in Germany," in *The Economics of Take-Off into Sustained Growth*, ed. W. W. Rostow (London: Macmillan, 1963), 95–118; Hans-Ulrich Wehler, *Das Deutsche Kaiserreich* (Göttingen: Vandenhoeck und Ruprecht, 1977), 24 and 41–59; Rainer Fremdling, "Railroads and German Economic Growth: A Leading Sector Analysis with a Comparison to the United States and Great Britain," *Journal of Economic History* 37 (1977): 583–604; Hans Rosenberg, "Wirtschaftskonjunktur, Gesellschaft, und Politik," in *Moderne deutsche Sozialgeschichte*, ed. Hans-Ulrich Wehler (Köln: Kiepenheuer und Witsch, 1976), 225–253.

3. Wolfgang Köllmann, "The Process of Urbanization in Germany at the Height of the Industrialization Period," *Journal of Contemporary History* 4 (1969): 62.

4. G. Hohorst, J. Kocka, and G. A. Ritter, *Sozialgeschichtliches Arbeitsbuch: Materialen zur Statistik des Kaiserreichs 1870–1914* (Munich: C. H. Beck, 1975), 19.

5. Wehler, *Das Deutsche Kaiserreich*, 60–140; Richard Evans, ed., *Society and Politics in Wilhelmine Germany* (New York: Barnes and Noble,

1978), 16–22; Wolfgang Mock, "Manipulation von oben oder Selbst-organisation an der Basis? Einige neuere Ansätze in der englischen Historiographie zur Geschichte des deutschen Kaiserreichs," *Historische Zeitschrift* 232 (1981): 358–375.

6. For a discussion of the radicalization of the labor movement as a result of the Anti-Socialist Law see Vernon L. Lidtke, *The Outlawed Party: Social Democracy in Germany, 1878–1890* (Princeton: Princeton University Press, 1966), 320–332.

7. For a brief discussion of the middle-class fear of the proletariat see Fritz Ringer, *The Decline of the German Mandarins: The German Academic Community, 1890–1933* (Cambridge, Mass.: Harvard University Press, 1969), 129; Fritz Stern, "The Political Consequences of the Unpolitical German," in *The Failure of Illiberalism: Essays on the Political Culture of Modern Germany* (Chicago: University of Chicago Press, 1975), 15; Guenther Roth, *The Social Democrats in Imperial Germany* (1963; reprint, New York: Arno Press, 1979), 85–101.

8. Vincent E. McHale and Eric A. Johnson, "Urbanization, Industrialization and Crime in Imperial Germany," *Social Science History* 1 (1976–77): 213. It should be pointed out, however, that the authors deal only with Prussia. Whether the rise in criminal activity was due to a real increase in the number of criminals or merely reflected an increase in the number of reported crimes remains unclear. It was probably a combination of the two.

9. Eduard Otto Mönkemöller, "Kriminalität," in *Handwörterbuch der sozialen Hygiene*, ed. A. Grotjahn and J. Kaup (Leipzig: F. C. W. Vogel, 1912), 1:687.

10. E. Fuld, "Das ruckfälliger Verbrechertum," *Deutsche Zeit- und Streit-Fragen* 14 (1885): 453–484; McHale and Johnson, "Urbanization, Industrialization and Crime," 212–214.

11. Eduard Otto Mönkemöller, "Kriminalität," 688.

12. Richard Evans, "Prostitution, State and Society in Imperial Germany," *Past and Present*, no. 70 (1976): 106–107.

13. Ibid., 108.

14. James S. Roberts, "Der Alkoholkonsum deutscher Arbeiter im 19. Jahrhundert," *Geschichte und Gesellschaft* 6 (1980): 226.

15. Ibid., 237.

16. Ibid., 232; Germany, Reichskommission, Internationale Hygiene-Ausstellung, Dresden, 1930–31, *Die Entwicklung des deutschen Gesundheitswesens* (Berlin: Arbeitgemeinschaft sozialhygienischer Reichsfachverbände, 1931), 18; Alfred Grotjahn, "Alkoholismus," in *Handwörterbuch der sozialen Hygiene*, 1:14. The most important pre-twentieth-century temperance organization was the Deutscher Verein gegen

Mißbrauch geistiger Getränke (German Association Against the Misuse of Alcoholic Beverages), founded in 1883.

17. Ludwig Meyer, "Die Zunahme der Geisteskrankheiten," *Deutsche Rundschau* (1885): 83; Alexander K. von Oettingen, *Die Moralstatistik in ihrer Bedeutung für eine Sozialethik*, 3d ed. (Erlangen: A. Deichert, 1882), 671; Arthur von Fircks, *Bevölkerung und Bevölkerungspolitik* (Leipzig: C. L. Hirschfeld, 1898), 116.

18. Schallmayer, *Vererbung und Auslese*, 1st. ed., 187–189; Eduard Otto Mönkemöller, "Selbstmord," in *Handwörterbuch der sozialen Hygiene*, 2:376.

19. Germany, Kaiserliches Statistisches Amt, *Statistisches Jahrbuch für das Deutsche Reich* (Berlin: Heymann, 1907), 64; Alfred Grotjahn, "Krankenhauswesen," in *Handwörterbuch der sozialen Hygiene*, 2:643.

20. The *soziale Frage* was born out of the contradiction between utopian social and political ideals (e.g., transcendence of class-conflict, the "unpolitical" state which stands above class interests) and the social and economic reality (a class society with class conflict) unleashed by Germany's industrial revolution. For a whole series of humanitarian, ethical, economic, military, and above all, political reasons, German social theorists believed it necessary to secure the (mythical) social harmony said to have been destroyed by economic liberalism and the process of industrialization. Albert Müssiggang, *Die soziale Frage in der historischen Schule der deutschen Nationalökonomie* (Tübingen: J. C. B. Mohr, 1968), 4. Müssiggang's book contains an extensive bibliography of both primary and secondary sources dealing with the social question.

21. See, for example, Adolf Wagner, *Rede über die soziale Frage* (Berlin: Wiegandt und Grieben, 1872); Gustav Schmoller, "Die soziale Frage und der preussische Staat," in *Quellen zur Geschichte der sozialen Frage in Deutschland*, 2d ed., Quellensammlung zur Kulturgeschichte, vol. 9, ed. Ernst Schraepler (Göttingen: Musterschmidt, 1964), 2:62–66; Friedrich Naumann, "Christlich-Sozial," in *Quellen zur Geschichte der soziale Frage*, 2:79–84; Ringer, *The Decline of the German Mandarins*, 145–147.

22. Müssigang, *Die soziale Frage*, 133.

23. In employing the word "organicism" to describe Marx's social theories I am following the philosopher of history Maurice Mandelbaum's definition of the term. Organicism refers "to the doctrine that human thought and action are invariably dependent upon the forms of organizations of social institutions." See Mandelbaum's *History, Man, and Reason: A Study in Nineteenth Century Thought* (Baltimore: The Johns Hopkins University Press, 1971), 170.

24. Ringer, *The Decline of the German Mandarins*, 146.

25. Ibid., 147.

26. James S. Roberts, *Drink, Temperance and the Working Class in Nine-teenth-Century Germany* (Boston: Allen & Unwin, 1984), 64.

27. For a discussion of the attitudes and prejudices of the Bildungsbürgertum see Klaus Vondung, ed., *Das wilhelminische Bildungsbürgertum: Zur Sozialgeschichte seiner Ideen* (Göttingen: Van-denhoeck und Ruprecht, 1976); Stern, "The Political Consequences of the Unpolitical German."

28. Vondung, *Das wilhelminische Bildungsbürgertum*, 26.

29. Ibid., 67–69.

30. Stern, "The Political Consequences of the Unpolitical German," passim; Roberts, *Drink, Temperance and the Working Class*, 55–56. The general cultural outlook of the Bildungsbürgertum is very evident in the German Association for the Prevention of Alcohol Abuse. The Associa-tion's attempt to project the cultural and moral values of its members onto society, its belief that it stood "above politics, as the guardians and purveyors of objective truth," and its desire to increase Germany's in-dustrial efficiency in order to make the Reich more competitive, are all remarkably similar to the aims of the German Society for Race Hygiene.

31. Baader and Schultz, eds., *Medizin und Nationalsozialismus*, 64.

32. Claudia Huerkamp, "Ärzte und Professionalisierung in Deutsch-land: Überlegungen zum Wandel des Arztberufs im 19. Jahrhundert," *Geschichte und Gesellschaft* 6 (1980): 366–367.

33. Eduard Seidler, "Der politische Standort des Arztes im zweiten Kaiserreich," in *Medizin, Naturwissenschaft, Technik und das zweite Kaiser-reich*, 91; Hans-Georg Güse and Norbert Schmacke, *Psychiatrie zwischen bürgerlicher Revolution und Faschismus* (Hamburg: Athenäum, 1976), 2:345–356; Godwin Jeschal, *Politik und Wissenschaft deutscher Ärzte im Ersten Weltkrieg*, Würzburger medizinhistorische Forschungen, Bd. 13 (1977), 21–22. There are, of course, many notable exceptions to this generalization concerning the political attitude of physicians; Rudolf Virchow is perhaps the most obvious one. Baader and Schultz, eds., *Medizin und Nationalsozialismus*, 56–60. It should be noted, however, that Baader and Schultz's discussion of the political attitude of physi-cians is limited to the First World War.

34. Seidler, "Der politische Standort," 87.

35. For a discussion of the health reform movement see Erwin H. Ackerknecht, "Beiträge zur Geschichte der Medizinalreform von 1848," *Archiv für Geschichte der Medizin* 25 (1932): 61–109, 112–183; Rosen, "Die Entwicklung der sozialen Medizin," in *Seminar: Medi-zin, Gesellschaft, Geschichte. Beitrage zur Entwicklungsgeschichte der Medizinsoziologe*, ed. Hans-Ulrich Deppe and Michael Regus (1975), 99–102.

36. Rosen, "Die Entwicklung der sozialen Medizin," 99–102.

37. George Rosen, *A History of Public Health* (New York: M. D. Publications, 1958), 225.

38. Although the reformers' hopes for a full-fledged public health program were not realized until the last quarter of the century, a "more limited program of sanitary reform" was undertaken in the years immediately following the defeat of the revolution. Ibid., 257; Gunter Mann, "Führende deutsche Hygieniker des 19. Jahrhunderts: Eine Übersicht," in *Städte-, Wohnungs- und Kleidungshygiene des 19. Jahrhunderts in Deutschland,* ed. Walter Artelt et. al. (Stuttgart: Ferdinand Enke, 1969), 7.

39. Stephan L. Chorover, *From Genesis to Genocide: The Meaning of Human Nature and the Power of Behavior Control* (Cambridge: MIT Press, 1979), 78.

40. Ackerknecht, "Beiträge zur Geschichte der Medizinalreform," 91.

41. Gerd Göckenjan, *Kurieren und Staat machen. Gesundheit und Medizin in der bürgerlichen Welt* (Frankfurt am Main: Suhrkamp, 1985), 240.

42. Rosen, *A History of Public Health,* 44; Seidler, "Der ˙politische Standort," 91–92; Eulner, "Hygiene als akademisches Fach," in *Städte-, Wohnungs- und Kleidungshygiene,* 18. Whereas academic medical researchers in the 1880s and 1890s undoubtedly enjoyed a very comfortable standard of living and a high measure of social prestige (partly owing to their position as civil servants), evidence suggests that at least some private practitioners were complaining about hard economic times. While the general practitioner was hardly on the brink of starvation, a general increase in the number of students studying medicine as well as the introduction of Bismarck's health insurance legislation made it more difficult for physicians without a field of specialization to secure their bourgeois life-style. In later years, as physicians became more financially dependent on the private insurance companies managing German health care, their economic situation became worse. For a discussion of the psychological and economic effects of Bismarck's health insurance laws on German physicians, see Robert J. Waldinger, "The High Priests of Nature: Medicine in Germany, 1883–1933" (B.A. thesis, Harvard University, 1973); Chorover, *From Genesis to Genocide,* 79; Huerkamp, "Ärzte und Professionalisierung in Deutschland," 367.

43. The recognition that social utility was a prerequisite for the professional prestige of the physician can be seen in the statement of one perceptive doctor in 1870—a time when the new developments in medicine had barely made an impact upon the professional fortunes of medical practitioners. "Only to the degree to which physicians elevate themselves above writing prescriptions and, as scientists and citizens, know how to render themselves useful and indispensable to society and state, will they receive the prize of public recognition still withheld from them." Göckenjan, *Kurieren und Staat,* 318.

44. Rosen, *A History of Public Health*, 166.

45. Germany, Reichsgesundheitsamt, *Das Reichsgesundheitsamt 1876–1926* (Berlin: Julius Springer, 1926), 6; Eulner, "Hygiene als akademisches Fach," 22.

46. Rosen, *A History of Public Health*, 167.

47. Eulner, "Hygiene als akademisches Fach," 19.

48. The role of physicians in the Third Reich will be discussed briefly in the Epilogue.

49. For a discussion of Alfred Grotjahn and the rise of social hygiene see Rosen, "Die Entwicklung der sozialen Medizin," 109–114. As will be demonstrated in chap. 4, social hygiene and eugenics do have much in common, and were not incompatible strategies for "improving national health." Until recently there has been a tendency in the literature dealing with the history of social medicine to view social hygiene as a unambiguously progressive discipline in contrast to the racist and reactionary eugenics movement. Recently, more critical studies of the history of social hygiene have revealed that it was greatly influenced by the concerns and rhetoric of eugenics. On this point see, for example, Paul Weindling, "Soziale Hygiene: Eugenik und medizinische Praxis— Der Fall Alfred Grotjahn," *Das Argument: Jahrbuch für kritische Medizin* (1984): 6–20. During the Weimar years Grotjahn was active in the Social Democratic party of Germany, and as such is an exception to the more common "apolitical" German physician.

50. Erwin H. Ackerknecht, *A Short History of Psychiatry*, 2d ed., trans. S. Wolff (New York and London: Hafner, 1968), 82.

51. A partial list of the available literature discussing the importance of heredity as an etiological factor in insanity is given in the bibliography to K. Grassman's article, "Kritische Ueberblick über die gegenwärtige Lehre von der Erblichkeit der Psychosen," *Allgemeine Zeitschrift für Psychiatrie* 52 (1896): 960–1022. With regard to the role assigned to heredity in epilepsy see Oscar Aronsohn, *Ueber Heredität bei Epilepsie* (Berlin: Wilhelm Axt, 1894). In addition, the etiological significance of the hereditary disposition for tuberculosis was also stressed in Germany's leading medical journals at this time. See, for example, M. Wahl, "Über den gegenwärtigen Stand der Erblichkeitsfrage in der Lehre von der Tuberculose," *Deutsche medizinische Wochenschrift* (1885), no. 1: 3–5, no. 3: 36–38, no. 4: 34–36, no. 5: 69–71, no. 6: 88–90. One institutional study available to physicians was "Über die Vererbung von Geisteskrankheiten nach Beobachtung in preussischen Irrenanstalten," *Jahrbuch für Psychiatrie und Neurologie* 1 (1879): 65–66.

52. George M. Beard was a specialist of sorts in the fields of electrotherapy and disorders of the nervous system. For a discussion of

Beard see, Charles E. Rosenberg, "George M. Beard and American Nervousness," *Bulletin of the History of Medicine* 36 (1962):245–259, reprinted in Rosenberg, *No Other Gods: On Science and American Social Thought* (Baltimore: The Johns Hopkins University Press, 1976), 98–108; Francis G. Gosling, "American Nervousness: A Study in American Medicine and Social Values in the Gilded Age, 1870–1900" (Ph.D. diss., University of Oklahoma, 1976).

53. George M. Beard, *American Nervousness: Its Causes and Consequences* (New York: G. P. Putnam's Sons, 1881), 16.

54. Beard, *American Nervousness,* Preface, iv. Beard was very conscious of Germany's overall scientific and medical superiority. He felt that history might, however, demonstrate that Europe had something to learn from America.

55. The term *erbliche Belastung* should be thought of as a hereditary disposition to some disease or disorder. Belastung literally means burden or handicap. Those who were "tainted"—people victimized by their own inferior disposition—were indeed burdened or handicapped, and it was a handicap that was impossible to overcome. For use of the word in German medical literature see Otto Binswanger, *Die Pathologie und Therapie der Neurasthenie: Vorlesungen für Studierende und Aerzte* (Jena: Gustav Fischer, 1896); Richard Freiherr von Krafft-Ebing, *Über gesunde und kranke Nerven* (Tübingen: Laupp'schen Buchhandlung, 1885); Leopold Löwenfeld, *Pathologie und Therapie der Neurasthenie und Hysterie* (Wiesbaden: J. F. Bergmann, 1894); Paul Julius Möbius, *Die Nervosität* (Leipzig: J. J. Weber, 1882). Other terms used to describe the same phenomenon include neuropathic disposition, neuropathic diathesis, nervous constitution, nervous taint, etc.

56. Möbius, *Die Nervosität,* 21.

57. Wilhelm Erb, *Über die wachsende Nervosität unserer Zeit* (Heidelberg: Universitäts-Buchdruckerei von J. Hörning, 1893), 22.

58. Löwenfeld, *Pathologie und Therapie der Neurasthenie und Hysterie,* 21–22.

59. Möbius, *Die Nervosität,* 31.

60. Some of the secondary sources on the origins of Morel's theory of degeneration and its impact on Western psychiatric thought include: Annemarie Wettley, "Zur Problemgeschichte der 'dégénérescence,'" *Sudhoffs Archiv* 43 (1959): 193–212; Wettley, "Der Entartungsbegriff und seine geistigen Abzweigungen in der Psychopathologie des 19. und 20. Jahrhunderts," *Jahrbuch für Psychologie* 6 (1958–59): 279–285; Wettley, "Entartung und Erbsünde: Der Einfluß des medizinischen Entartungsbegriffs auf den literarischen Naturalismus," *Hochland* 51 (1958–59): 348–358; Peter Burgener, *Die Einflüsse des zeitgenossichen Denkens in*

Morels Begriff der "dégénérescence," Zürcher medizingeschichtliche Abhandlungen, no. 16 (Zürich: Juris, 1964); Ruth Friedlander, "Benedict Augustin Morel and the Development of the Theory of 'dégénérescence'" (Ph.D. diss., University of San Francisco, 1973); Ackerknecht, *A Short History of Psychiatry,* chap. 7.

61. Wettley, "Zur Problemgeschichte der 'dégénéresence,' " 195-196.

62. Wettley, "Der Entartungsbegriff," 280-281; Ackerknecht, *A Short History of Psychiatry,* 56.

63. Möbius, *Über Entartung* (Wiesbaden: J. F. Bergmann, 1900), 95-96, 99.

64. Richard Freiherr von Krafft-Ebing, "Nervosität und neurasthenische Zustände," *Specielle Pathologie und Therapie,* ed. Hermann Nothnagel (Vienna: Alfred Holder, 1899), vol. 2, pt. 2:5.

65. For a discussion of Lombroso and the relationship of his ideas to the origins of modern criminology, see Robert A. Nye, "Heredity or Milieu: The Foundations of Modern European Criminological Theory," *Isis* 67 (1976): 335-381.

66. Hans Kurella, *Naturgeschichte des Verbrechers* (Stuttgart: Ferdinand Enke, 1893).

67. See, for example, Robert Gaupp, "Über den heutigen Stand der Lehre von 'geborenen Verbrecher,'" *Monatsschrift für Kriminalpsychologie und Strafrechtsreform* 1 (1904): 33; Paul Näcke, "Über den Wert der sogenannten Degenerationszeichen," *Monatsschrift für Kriminalpsychologie und Strafrechtsreform* 1 (1904); 108; and Gustav Aschaffenburg, *Crime and Its Repression,* trans. Adalbert Albrecht (Boston: Little, Brown and Co., 1913), 177.

68. Gaupp, "Über den heutigen Stand der Lehre von 'geborenen Verbrecher,'" 32.

69. Ibid., 31.

70. *Constitutionspathologie* or *Constitutionslehre* represented, at least in part, a movement away from Virchow's *anatomischer Gedanke* (anatomical perspective) among German pathologists beginning around 1890. Whereas Virchow stressed the localization of disease and identified its cause as some external stimulus, the originators of the Constitutionslehre (Ottomar Rosenbach, Ferdinand Hueppe, and Friedrich Martius) reacted against Virchow's limited perspective. Pathological anatomy proved impotent as a viable interpretive framework for a whole series of so-called functional ailments and constitutional diseases. Defenders of the Constitutionslehre minimized the importance of Virchow's external stimulus as the etiological factor in disease and focused on the individual's overall bodily constitution. Rather than investigate the disease, pathologists such as Martius found more promise in a

careful examination of diseased individuals (including their forefathers and descendants). As Henry E. Sigerist has pointed out, the shift in medical thinking in favor of the constitution formed the basis for eugenic thought. See Henry E. Sigerist, "Das Bild des Menschen in der modernen Medizin," *Neue Blätter für den Sozialismus* 1 (1930); 102. Martius himself was an enthusiastic supporter of the German eugenics movement and a member of the Deutsche Gesellschaft für Rassenhygiene. For a discussion see Rainer Krügel, *Friedrich Martius und der konstitutionelle Gedanke*, Marburger Schriften zur Medizingeschichte, Bd. 11 (Frankfurt am Main: Peter Lang, 1984); Paul Diepgen, "Krankheitswesen und Krankheitsursachen in der speculativen Pathologie des 19. Jahrhunderts," *Sudhoffs Archiv* 18 (1926); 302–327; Paul Diepgen, *Geschichte der Medizin*, 2:2 (Berlin: Walter de Gruyter and Co., 1955); 138–144.

71. Wahl, "Über den gegenwärtigen Stand," 5.

72. Möbius, *Die Nervosität*, 27–28.

73. Moriz Kende, *Die Entartung des Menschengeschlechts, ihre Ursachen und die Mittel zu ihrer Bekämpfung* (Halle: Carl Marhold, 1901), 36–48.

74. The importance of natural selection for evolutionary theory was discussed in the works of several German-speaking eugenicists and their supporters. See Schallmayer, *Vererbung und Auslese*, 1st ed., p. 3; Alfred Ploetz, *Die Tüchtigkeit unsrer Rasse und der Schutz der Schwachen. Ein Versuch über Rassenhygiene und ihr Verhältnis zu den humanen Idealen, besonders zum Sozialismus* (Berlin: Gustav Fischer, 1895), 16; August Forel, *The Sexual Question*, 2d ed. trans. C. F. Marshal (New York: Physicians' and Surgeons' Book Company, 1924), 42; Heinrich E. Ziegler, *Die Vererbungslehre in der Biologie und in der Soziologie* (Jena: Gustav Fischer, 1918), 165.

75. For an excellent treatment of natural selection as metaphor, its problems and its appeal, see Robert Young, "Darwin's Metaphor: Does Nature Select?" *Monist* 55 (1971); 442–503.

76. For a discussion of the influence of Greg, Wallace, and Galton on Darwin's views concerning the role of natural selection in human and social evolution see Lyndsay Farrall, "The Origins and Growth of the English Eugenics Movement" (Ph.D. diss., Indiana University, 1970), 11–27.

77. John C. Greene, "Darwin as a Social Evolutionist," *Journal of the History of Biology* 10 (1977); 11.

78. Charles Darwin, *Descent of Man and Selection in Relation to Sex*, 2d ed. (1876; reprint, New York: The Modern Library, n.d.), 504.

79. Ibid., 507.

80. Ibid., 918–919.

81. William M. Montgomery, "Germany," in *The Comparative Reception of Darwin,* ed. Thomas F. Glick (Austin: University of Texas Press, 1974), 81.

82. Ibid., 83.

83. Schallmayer did not become familiar with Weismann's work until after the publication of his first short treatise. See chap. 3.

84. One historian of science has even gone so far as to suggest that in the last revised edition of Darwin's *Origin,* the title was misleading. It would have been more appropriate had it read: "On the Origin of Species by Means of Natural Selection and All Sorts of Other Things." Young, "Darwin's Metaphor," 496–497.

85. Darwin's Lamarckian influences can most clearly be seen in his somewhat less well-known work, *The Variation of Animals and Plants Under Domestication* (New York: O. Judd and Co., 1868).

86. August Weismann, "On Heredity," in *Essays Upon Heredity and Kindred Problems,* ed. Edward Poulton, Selmar Schönland, and Arthur Shipley (Oxford: Clarendon Press, 1889), 72.

87. Ibid., 78.

88. Ibid., Preface and 69; also see Fredrick Churchill, "August Weismann and a Break from Tradition," *Journal of the History of Biology* 1 (1968): 101.

89. Weismann was quick to point out that neither direct observation nor experiment demonstrated the inheritance of acquired characteristics. The Freiburg embryologist concluded with DuBois Reymond that "the hereditary transmission of acquired characters remains an unintelligible hypothesis, which is only deduced from the facts which it attempts to explain." Weismann, "On Heredity," 82.

90. Ibid., 90.

91. Ibid., 86.

92. August Weismann, *Vorträge über Deszendenztheorie,* 2d ed. (Jena: Gustav Fischer, 1904), 2:123–125.

93. Alfred Kelly, *The Descent of Darwin: The Popularization of Darwinism in Germany, 1860–1914* (Chapel Hill: University of North Carolina Press, 1981), 5.

94. Ibid., 23, 130.

95. Ibid., 22.

96. For a full discussion of Haeckel's monism see Gasman, *The Scientific Origins of National Socialism.*

97. I have used the following English translation: Ernst Haeckel, *The History of Creation: Or the Development of the Earth and Its Inhabitants by the Action of Natural Causes,* trans. and revised by E. Ray Lankester (London: Henry S. King and Co., 1876), 1:120.

98. Ibid., 277.

99. For a discussion of Spencer's "law of progress," see his famous 1857 article, "Progress: Its Law and Cause," reprinted in his *Essays Scientific, Political and Speculative* (New York: D. Appelton and Co., 1891), 8–62.

100. Haeckel, *The History of Creation*, 1:172.

101. Ibid., 172–173.

102. Ibid., 174.

103. In my use of the term I am following John Greene's definition of social Darwinism as "the belief that competition between individuals, tribes, nations, and races has been an important, if not the chief, engine of progress in human history." See Greene, "Darwin as a Social Evolutionist," 26. At least two historians adhere to a similar periodization of social Darwinism. Kelly, *The Descent of Darwin*, chap. 6; Zmarzlik, "Sozialdarwinismus in Deutschland," 246–273.

104. Rosenberg, "Wirtschaftskonjunktur," 233.

105. Kelly, *The Descent of Darwin*, 105–106.

106. Hermann W. Siemens, *Die biologischen Grundlagen der Rassenhygiene und der Bevölkerungspolitik* (Munich: J. F. Lehmann, 1917), 10.

107. There were, of course, some second generation social Darwinists who did not become involved with eugenics. The so-called social anthropologist Otto Ammon (1862–1916), and the deputy business director of the Organization of German Industrialists, Alexander Tille (1866–1912), are two of the most important such figures. For a discussion of Ammon's racial anthropology see chap. 4.

2: THE RATIONALIZATION
OF HEREDITY AND SELECTION

1. Although Schallmayer was baptized Friedrich Wilhelm, he always used the first name Wilhelm.

2. Max von Gruber, "Wilhelm Schallmayer," *Archiv für Rassen- und Gesellschafts-Biologie* (hereafter cited as *ARGB*) 14 (1922): 55. Information also obtained from a 1977 interview I had with Wilhelm Schallmayer's son, Friedrich Schallmayer, in Karlsruhe, West Germany.

3. Otto Schallmayer, "Wilhelm Schallmayer," *Akademischer Gesangverein* (1919 or 1920): 1.

4. Ibid. Schallmayer considered militarism *kulturfeindlich*. He spoke out against it in many of his articles and works. Yet, as we shall see, he was not totally free of the militaristic/imperialistic spirit of the day.

5. Interview with Friedrich Schallmayer. Unpublished *Studiumzeugnisse* in the possession of F. Schallmayer. Also see Fritz Lenz, "Wilhelm Schallmayer," *Münchener medizinische Wochenschrift* 66 (1919): 1295.

6. For secondary literature on Wilhelm Wundt, see Edwin G. Boring, *A History of Experimental Psychology* (New York and London: D. Appleton and Co., 1929), 310–344; G. Stanley Hall, *Founders of Modern Psychology* (New York: D. Appleton and Co., 1912), 311–458; Rudolf Eisler, *Wilhelm Wundts Philosophie und Psychologie* (Leipzig: Johann Ambrosius Barth, 1902); Willy Nef, *Die Philosophie Wilhelm Wundts* (Leipzig: Felix Meiner, 1923). Wundt defined the relationship between philosophy and the other sciences in the following manner: "Philosophie ist die allgemeine Wissenschaft, welche die durch die Einzelwissenschaften vermittelten Erkenntnisse zu einem widerspruchslosen System zu vereinigen und die von der Wissenschaft benutzten allgemeinen Methoden und Voraussetzungen des Erkennens auf ihre Prinzipien zurückzuführen hat." Nef, *Die Philosophie Wilhelm Wundts,* 14. Nef is quoting from Wundt's *Einleitung in die Philosophie,* 2d ed. (Leipzig: W. Engelmann, 1902), 19.

7. Unpublished *Studiumzeugnisse.* In the summer of 1880 Schallmayer attended two of Wundt's courses: Psychologische Gesellschaft and Psychologie I.

8. Lenz, "Schallmayer," 1295; Gruber, "Schallmayer," 55.

9. For a discussion of the *Kathedersozialisten* see Vernon Lidtke, *The Outlawed Party,* 62–64.

10. See Schallmayer, "Rassenhygiene und Sozialismus," *Die neue Zeit* 25 (1906–07): 735. Gruber, in his obituary of Schallmayer, speaks of a *monistisch-demokratisch* (monistic-democratic) *international-pazifistischer Radikalismus* (pacifistic-radicalism) which characterized the latter's youth, and from which he "was never quite free." Gruber, "Schallmayer," 53–54. There is a remarkable parallel between the political outlook of Schallmayer and that of the British eugenicist Karl Pearson. Pearson also seemed to be inclined toward a form of non-Marxist state socialism with social imperialist overtones which closely resembled the views of Schallmayer. For a discussion of Pearson see Daniel J. Kevles, *In the Name of Eugenics: Genetics and the Uses of Human Heredity* (New York: Knopf, 1985), 21–24.

11. In Germany a person who has earned a medical degree does not automatically receive the title "doctor" as is the case in the United States. It is necessary to write a dissertation, usually on some clinical subject, to obtain the title. Although a physician can legally practice medicine without the title, there is definite social and professional pressure to secure it.

12. There is still much mystery surrounding the relationship between

von Gudden and Ludwig II (1845–1886). After a regent was appointed, Ludwig apparently suffered an even more severe case of paranoia. He was immediately brought to Schloß Berg at Starnberg Lake on June 10, 1886, and placed in von Gudden's care. Three days later, allegedly in an attempt to win the monarch's trust, von Gudden accompanied Ludwig to the lake where a fight between the two of them ensued. Von Gudden was probably knocked unconscious and drowned. Ludwig's body was also found in the water. For a biographical sketch of von Gudden, see Emil Kraepelin, "Bernhard von Gudden," *Münchener medizinische Wochenschrift* 33 (1886): 577–580 and 603–607.

13. Interview with F. Schallmayer.

14. This evidence seems to contradict Loren Graham's assertion that Schallmayer was a radical democrat. Graham, "Science and Values," 1136.

15. See Kraepelin, "Von Gudden," 607.

16. Schallmayer, "Die Nahrungsverweigerung und die übrigen Störungen der Nahrungsaufnahme bei Geisteskranken" (Med. Diss., Munich, 1885).

17. Lenz, "Schallmayer," 1295.

18. Wilhelm Schallmayer, "Einführung in die Rassehygiene," in *Ergebnisse der Hygiene, Bakteriologie, Immunitätsforschung und experimentalen Therapie,* ed. W. Weichards, (Berlin: J. Springer, 1917), 2:524. The four Social Democratic journals which reviewed Schallmayer's text are the *Volkswille* (Hannover), *Hamburger Echo, Volkstimme* (Magdeburg), and *Die neue Zeit* (theoretical organ of the SPD).

19. Schallmayer, *Die drohende physische Entartung der Culturvölker,* 2d ed. (Berlin and Neuwied: Heuser, 1895), 1. I have been unable to obtain a copy of the first edition. Judging, however, from the reviews of the first edition, the second edition varied little, if at all, from the 1891 printing. It seems probable that Schallmayer read Haeckel's *History of Creation,* although he does not cite him in the text. There are so many similarities between the two authors that sheer coincidence is unlikely. See Haeckel, *History of Creation,* 1:25–27. He not only cites Haeckel's *History of Creation* in his later *Vererbung und Auslese* but also credits Haeckel with contributing both directly and indirectly to eugenics in Germany. See Schallmayer, "Ernst Haeckel und die Eugenik," in *Was Wir Ernst Haeckel Verdanken,* ed. Heinrich Schmidt (Leipzig: Unesma, 1914), 2:368.

20. Schallmayer, *Die drohende physische Entartung,* 1–3.

21. Ibid., 3.

22. Ibid., 5.

23. Ibid., 5–6.

24. Ibid., 6.

25. Ibid., 6.

26. Ibid., 10.

27. Ibid., 12–13.

28. Ibid., 13.

29. Ibid., 15–16.

30. Ibid., 7–8.

31. The term "pauper idiot" is used by Nikolas Rose in his article, "The Psychological Complex: Mental Measurement and Social Administration," *Ideology and Consciousness* 5 (1979): 39. Rose also discusses the notion of degenerate stock which manifests itself as various forms of deviant behavior (e.g. criminality, immorality, unemployability, etc.).

32. Schallmayer, *Die drohende physische Entartung,* 17–18.

33. Ibid., 18.

34. Schallmayer, *Vererbung und Auslese. Grundriß der Gesellschaftsbiologie und der Lehre vom Rassedienst,* 3d ed. (Jena: Gustav Fischer, 1918), 338–339. On these pages Schallmayer outlines the eugenicist Max von Gruber's plan to "reform" the German inheritance law.

35. Ribot, founder of the *Revue philosophique* and professor at the Collège de France, dedicated himself to the establishment of a psychology free from any metaphysical underpinnings. The influence of Taine, Spencer, and Wundt is evident in his works. More specifically, Ribot was concerned with the relationship between normal and pathological behavior. Many of the ideas set out in his *L'hérédité,* including the inheritance of all mental traits, was undoubtedly colored by the works of Galton and Darwin, both of whom he cites. For a brief discussion of Ribot see Linda L. Clark, *Social Darwinism in France* (University: University of Alabama Press, 1984), 42–44.

36. Ribot, *Heredity: A Psychological Study of Its Phenomena, Laws, Causes, and Consequences* (New York: D. Appleton & Co., 1875), 305. Published in French, 1873.

37. Ibid., 289–290.

38. For a background of late nineteenth century views concerning heredity see Frederick Churchill, "Rudolf Virchow and the Pathologist's Criteria for the Inheritance of Acquired Characteristics," *Journal of the History of Medicine* 31 (1976): 117–148.

39. Schallmayer, *Die drohende physische Entartung,* 11–12.

40. In Part II of his treatise, Schallmayer discusses the need to compile genealogies and health statistics in order to determine in advance not only who should be prevented from marrying but also whether a person's prospective marriage partner was, eugenically speaking, a good catch.

41. Schallmayer, *Die drohende physische Entartung,* 9.

42. For a discussion of why Schallmayer employed the term Rassehygiene instead of Rassenhygiene, see chap. 3.

43. Schallmayer, *Die drohende physische Entartung*, 9–10.

44. Ibid., 10.

45. For a discussion of the socialization process of the German education system, see Wehler, *Das Deutsche Kaiserreich*, 125–126.

46. Schallmayer, *Die drohende physische Entartung*, 20.

47. Ibid. "Wir aber schmälern nach Verschwenderart dieses Fideicommiss, das wir ihnen unverkürzt schuldig sind."

48. Ibid., 23.

49. Ibid., 25.

50. Ibid., 25–27. For those with no diseases, it would suffice to turn the cards in every five to ten years, at which point they would be issued a new card. To make sure that the local offices and central ministry were aware of all cases of an illness, every physician was expected to notify officials at the office weekly or monthly of all entries made on their patients' health cards. This would assure that if a patient did not turn in his or her card to the physician (as was demanded), the local office would still have a record of the person's illness.

51. Ibid., 28.

52. Ibid., 30–31.

53. Ibid., 32.

54. Ibid., 33.

55. Ibid., 33.

56. Schallmayer later devoted much attention to this subject and wrote a separate article on it. See Schallmayer, "Generative Ethik," *ARGB* 6 (1909): 199–231.

57. Schallmayer, *Die drohende physische Entartung*, 34–35.

58. This was largely owing to the *Gewerbeordnung* of 1869 which made medicine a "free trade" subject to the laws of supply and demand, the introduction of Bismarck's health insurance laws, and the increased number of physicians relative to the population.

59. Schallmayer, *Die drohende physische Entartung*, 36.

60. For a discussion of the privileges and status enjoyed by the German bureaucracy see J. Röhl, "Beamtenpolitik in wilhelminischen Deutschland," in *Das kaiserliche Deutschland*, ed. M. Stürmer (Düsseldorf: Droste, 1970), 387–411; Lysbeth W. Muncy, *The Junker in the Prussian Administration, 1888–1914* (New York: Howard Fertig, 1970); and Ringer, *The Decline of the German Mandarins*.

61. At the time, Schallmayer believed, many physicians would not see the advantages of becoming civil servants, but this would change. "Bei dem rapiden Anwachsen der ärztlichen Konkurrenz droht das Einkommen und auch das Aussehen der Ärzte in solchem Grade zu sinken, dass vielleicht in nicht sehr ferner Zeit die Mehrzahl der Ärzte es freudig begrüssen würde, zu der relativ gesicherten Stellung und dem

Ansehen von Staatsbeamten zu gelingen." Schallmayer, *Über die drohende physische Entartung*, 37. Concerning free competition among physicians, Schallmayer had the following to say: "Ich will hier auf die demoralisirende Wirkung einer zu grossen freien Konkurrenz nicht näher eingehen. Je mehr die Konkurrenz wächst, desto unpassender wird die Bezeichnung Kollege, welche nur bei ausschließlich amtlicher Stellung der Ärzte zu ihrem vollen Rechte käme." Ibid., 37.

62. See for example the anonymous book review, "Ueber die drohende körperliche Entartung der Culturmenschheit und die Verstaatlichung des ärztlichen Standes." *Münchener medizinische Wochenschrift* 27 (1892): 478–480; and H. Knieke, "Die Verstaatlichung des Aerztewesens," *Politisch-anthropologische Revue* 2 (1903–1904): 402–409.

63. Knieke, "Die Verstaatlichung," 402.

64. After the founding of the Reich, the national health office was made a part of the Kultusministerium. It was later to come under the jurisdiction of the Ministerium des Innern (Ministry of Interior).

65. Schallmayer, "Ein Medizinalministerium," *Das neue Jahrhundert* 1 (1898): 393.

66. Schallmayer, *Die drohende physische Entartung*, 35.

67. Ibid., 35.

3: THE KRUPP COMPETITION OF 1900 AND SCHALLMAYER'S AWARD WINNING TREATISE

1. The problem of and solution to degeneration was, however, discussed by Alfred Ploetz, the second co-founder of German eugenics, in his work, *Die Tüchtigkeit unsrer Rasse* published in 1895. Ploetz's book, the first treatise on *Rassenhygiene* as such, did not, however, receive widespread attention until after the Krupp competition of 1900.

2. From what he inherited from his father, his wife's wealth, and the money he saved during the time he worked as a practicing physician, Schallmayer was able to live comfortably as an independent scholar. His situation improved still further in 1903 after winning 10,000 marks in the Krupp Contest.

3. Apparently there is some confusion in the historical literature concerning just which Krupp sponsored the *Preisausschreiben* of 1900. Some historians have not bothered to tell their readers whether it was Alfred Krupp or his son, Friedrich Alfred, who donated the money for

the contest. See Poliakov, *The Aryan Myth*, 294, and Zmarzlik, "Sozialdarwinismus in Deutschland," 264. Several scholars, following the incorrect lead provided by Conrad-Martius in *Utopien der Menschenzüchtung*, 74, wrongly believe the donor to have been Alfred Krupp. See Alfred Kelly, *The Descent of Darwin*, 107; Graham, "Science and Values," 1135; Gasman, *The Scientific Origins of National Socialism*, 148; Bolle, "Darwinismus und Zeitgeist," 166.

4. There is an enormous literature dealing with various aspects of the rise and legacy of the House of Krupp. Much of it, however, is not very recent or very critical. The best comprehensive work appears to be that William Manchester, *The Arms of Krupp* (Boston: Little, Brown and Co., 1968). Other family histories include Norbert Muhlen, *The Incredible Krupps. The Rise, Fall, and Comeback of Germany's Industrial Family* (New York: Henry Holt and Co., 1959), and Gert von Klass, *Krupps: The Story of an Industrial Empire*, trans. James Cleugh (London: Sidgwick and Jackson, 1954).

5. Muhlen, *The Incredible Krupps*, 3–24.

6. Ibid., 39–44. Also see Manchester, *The Arms of Krupp*, 63–93.

7. Muhlen, *The Incredible Krupps*, 49–50.

8. Manchester, *The Arms of Krupp*, 152–53.

9. Ibid., 152, 158; Muhlen, *The Incredible Krupps*, 59–62, 65; Joachim Schlacht, "Die Kruppsiedlungen—Wohnungsbau im Interesse eines Industriekonzerns," in *Kapitalistischer Städtebau*, ed. Hans G. Helms and Jörn Janssen (Neuwied and Berlin: Hermann Luchterhand, 1970), 95–111.

10. Muhlen, *The Incredible Krupps*, 65.

11. Manchester, *The Arms of Krupp*, 258–259. Allegedly the marine biologists Anton Dohrn and Otto Zacharias conceded that Krupp had collected thirty-three new species of marine animals.

12. Muhlen, *The Incredible Krupps*, 91. This version of the story is contested by Manchester who suggests that Krupp made the initial overture to Dohrn and that Dohrn, considering the Naples Station to be a place for professional biologists, wanted no part of Krupp.

13. Günter Wendel, *Die Kaiser-Wilhelm-Gesellschaft 1911–1914* (Berlin-East: Akademie, 1975), 47.

14. The famous Virchow-Haeckel debate took place in Munich on September 22, 1877. Virchow's entire address is reprinted in Rudolf Virchow, *The Freedom of Science in the Modern State*, 2d ed. (London: John Murray, 1878). For a discussion of the debate, see Kelly, *Descent of Darwin*, 58–61.

15. For a discussion of the early reception of Darwinism by German Social Democratic intellectuals, see Zmarzlik, "Sozialdarwinismus in Deutschland"; Bolle, "Darwinismus und Zeitgeist"; and especially

Hans-Josef Steinberg, *Sozialismus und deutsche Sozialdemokratie* (Bonn-Bad Godesberg: J. H. W. Dietz, 1976), 45–51.

16. Ernst Haeckel, *Freedom in Science and Teaching* (New York: D. Appleton, 1879), 90–93.

17. Ziegler to Haeckel, 4 October 1899, Ernst-Haeckel-Haus Jena, Best. A-Abt. 1 No n 0005. The correspondence between Krupp and Haeckel begins in 1901, and they apparently first met in August 1902. The anti-Social Democratic and pro-National Liberal intent behind the contest is clearly visible in a rambling *"Niederschrift"* written by Krupp in January 1900. Krupp-Archiv Essen, IX-d-244, and correspondence in III-D-159. I am indebted to Jeff Johnson, who provided me with his notes from the Krupp-Archiv.

18. Heinrich Ernst Ziegler, "Einleitung zu dem Sammelwerke Natur und Staat" in *Natur und Staat: Beiträge zur naturwissenschaftlichen Gesellschaftslehre* (Jena: Gustav Fischer, 1903), 1–2.

19. Ziegler, "Einleitung," 2–3.

20. Ibid., 4; Heinrich Ernst Ziegler, *Die Vererbungslehre in der Biologie und in der Soziologie* (Jena: Gustav Fischer, 1918), Vorwort, xiii-xiv; Wilhelm Schallmayer, *Vererbung und Auslese in ihrer soziologischen und politischen Bedeutung,* 2d ed. (Jena: Gustav Fischer, 1910), Vorwort, viii.

21. Ziegler, *Die Vererbungslehre,* Vorwort, xii.

22. Heinrich Ernst Ziegler, *Die Naturwissenschaft und die socialdemokratische Theorie, ihr Verhältnis dargelegt auf Grund der Werke von Darwin und Bebel* (Stuttgart: Ferdinand Enke, 1893), 23.

23. August Bebel, *Die Frau und der Sozialismus* (Frankfurt am Main: Marxistische Blätter, 1977), 10–11. Bebel states that Ziegler is "most probably" a National Liberal.

24. Karl Diehl, "Johannes Conrad," *Jahrbücher für Nationalökonomie und Statistik* 104 (1915), 757–758.

25. Ziegler, "Einleitung," 4.

26. Ibid., 7.

27. Ibid., 20.

28. Ibid., 21.

29. Ibid.

30. Ibid., 18.

31. Ibid.

32. Ibid., 19.

33. Ziegler, "Einleitung," 6.

34. Ibid., 15–16.

35. Ibid., 9.

36. Schallmayer, *Vererbung und Auslese,* 1st ed., 380–381.

37. Ibid., x.

38. Ibid., 3. For the intrusion of other mechanisms into Darwin's theory, see chap. 1.

39. Ibid.

40. Ibid., 95-96.

41. Ibid., 32.

42. For an excellent discussion of Neo-Lamarckism see Peter J. Bowler, *The Eclipse of Darwinism: Anti-Darwinian Evolution Theories in the Decades around 1900* (Baltimore: Johns Hopkins University Press, 1983), esp. chap. 4; Idem., *Evolution: The History of an Idea* (Berkeley, Los Angeles, London: University of California Press, 1984), 243-265.

43. A brief discussion of Davenport's scientific training is offered in Mark H. Haller, *Eugenics: Hereditarian Attitudes in American Thought* (New Brunswick: Rutgers University Press, 1983), 63-64; Kevles, *In the Name of Eugenics,* 50-51. The only *major* German eugenicists with a training in genetics were Fritz Lenz and Otmar Freiherr von Verschuer. Lenz attended Weismann's courses while the former was studying at Freiburg. Other genetically-trained biologists who were involved in the German eugenics movement during the Weimar years include Erwin Baur, Richard Goldschmidt, Carl Correns, and Heinrich Poll. Paul Weindling, "Weimar Eugenics: The Kaiser Wilhelm Institute for Anthropology, Human Heredity and Eugenics in Social Context," *Annals of Science* 42 (1985): 304.

44. Ibid., 63.

45. Ibid., 59.

46. Ibid., 62.

47. August Weismann, "On the Duration of Life," in *Essays Upon Heredity and Kindred Problems,* 9-10.

48. Schallmayer, *Vererbung und Auslese,* 1st ed., 236.

49. Ibid., 242.

50. Ibid., 89-94.

51. Ibid., 76.

52. Ibid., 214.

53. Otto Seeck, author of *Geschichte des Untergangs der antiken Welt* (reprint; Darmstadt: Wissenschaftliche Buchgesellschaft, 1966) was considered by Schallmayer to be part of a small, but expanding group of researchers who had come to view "history from the standpoint of biological selection." Also included in this group was Joseph Arthur Comte de Gobineau, Francis Galton, Théodule Armand Ribot, and Georges Vacher de Lapouge. See Schallmayer, *Vererbung und Auslese,* 1st ed., 181.

54. Schallmayer, *Vererbung und Auslese,* 1st ed., 185.

55. Ibid., 193-211.

56. Wilhelm Schallmayer, "Kultur und Entartung," *Monatsschrift für soziale Medizin und Hygiene* 1 (1906): 488. Using information from another author, Schallmayer argued that out of a sample of 387 Germans, 75 percent had a cranial capacity of over 1300 cc whereas of 108 Chinese, 92 percent had over 1300 cc. Whereas 8 percent of the white race had a cranial capacity of less than 1200 cc, only 2 percent of the yellow race measured less than 1200 cc. On this same point regarding the high intelligence of the Chinese see Wilhelm Schallmayer, "Die Erbentwicklung bei Völkern als theoretisches und praktisches Problem," *Menschheitsziele* (1907): 93.

57. Schallmayer, *Vererbung und Auslese*, 1st ed., 196−197 n. Schallmayer's high regard for the biological efficiency of the Chinese later became mixed with fear, as discussions of the "yellow peril" became more numerous in Germany after the turn of the century. See chap. 5.

58. Ibid., 245. "Nach den Grundsätzen, die sich aus der Descendenzlehre ableiten lassen, ist es also die höchste Aufgabe der inneren Politik, der sich alle andere Aufgaben unterzuordnen haben, innerhalb der Bevölkerung die Daseinsbedingungen so zu gestalten, wie es das Machtbedürfnis im internationalen Daseinskampf erfordert."

59. Ibid., 246−247.

60. Ibid., 247−248.

61. Ibid., 248.

62. Fritz Krupp committed suicide in 1902 after reports of his homosexual activities were leaked to the German press.

63. Schallmayer, "Auslese beim Menschen: Eine Erwiderung," *Zeitschrift für philosophische Kritik* 129 (1907): 143; Wilhelm Schallmayer, *Beiträge zu einer Nationalbiologie* (Jena: Hermann Constenoble, 1905), 251.

64. For a discussion of the German intellectuals' relationship to political parties, see chap. 1.

65. Schallmayer, *Vererbung und Auslese*, 1st ed., 368−375.

66. Ibid., 324.

67. Ibid., 373.

68. Ibid. Perhaps Schallmayer's clearest position on his views regarding meritocracy can be found in his article entitled, "Rassehygiene und Sozialismus," *Die neue Zeit* 25 (1906−07): 735. "Mein soziales Ideal ist eine Gesellschaftsordnung, die man als *Leistungsaristokratie* bezeichnen kann. Demokratisch und sozialistisch ist dieses Ideal insofern, als es die Forderung enthält, die äusseren Wettbewerbsbedingungen für die Jugend in jeder Hinsicht so viel wie nur irgend möglich gleich zu gestalten, dann aber die Personen, die unter den gleichen äusseren Wettbewerbsbedingungen mehr leisten, entsprechend besser zu stellen, an

Ehren, Einkommen und generativen Chancen; dies alles jedoch mit solchen Modificationen, daß dadurch die Gleichheit der äusseren Wettbewerbsbedingungen für die Jugend nicht beeinträchtigt wird." For a discussion of Pearson, see Kevles, *In the Name of Eugenics,* 24.

69. There was also another important category in Schallmayer's overall schema: *Bevölkerungspolitik* (population policy). This category will be discussed at length in chap. 5.

70. Schallmayer, *Vererbung und Auslese,* 1st ed., 297–298.

71. Ibid., 303.

72. Ibid., 90. In Germany the demand for mandatory sanctions in the area of negative eugenics grew louder during the stormy years of the late Weimar republic. The 1933 sterilization law ended this tradition of voluntarism once and for all. For more details, see the Epilogue.

73. Ibid., 338.

74. Ibid., 338–339.

75. Ibid., 354.

76. Ibid., 360–361. Schallmayer was referring to the attempt to pass eugenic legislation in the state of North Dakota. He praised an already existing law in Michigan that prohibited the mentally ill and "idiots" from marrying. This same statute also forced those who married while being infected with venereal disease to pay a heavy fine.

77. Ibid., 345–346.

78. Ibid., 346.

4: CONTINUITY AND CONTROVERSY

1. Some of the professional journals include *Zeitschrift für Sozialpolitik und Verwaltung, Deutsche Literaturzeitung, Naturwissenschaftliche Wochenschrift, Zeitschrift für Philosophie und philosophische Kritik, Archiv für die gesamte Psychologie, Münchener medizinische Wochenschrift, Archiv für Rassen- und Gesellschafts-Biologie, Hygienische Rundschau, Zeitschrift für Sexualwissenschaft, Jahrbücher für Nationalökonomie,* and the *Politsch-anthropologische Revue.* The *Frankfurter Zeitung* and *Der Tag* are the two newspapers containing reviews of the first edition of *Vererbung und Auslese;* the former was a highbrow paper, the latter was a social democratic publication. The arch-conservative journal referred to is the *Preussische Jahrbücher;* the socialist organs are *Die neue Zeit* and *Sozialistische Monatshefte.*

2. The term "social anthropology" as used in this chapter is radically different from its contemporary meaning. Today the term is used to denote the sub-discipline of anthropology which "aims at understanding and explaining the diversity of human behavior by a comparative

study of social relationships and processes over as wide a range of societies as possible." Raymond Firth, "Social Anthropology," *International Encyclopedia of the Social Sciences* (New York: Macmillan Co. and the Free Press, 1968), 1−2:320−324.

3. One of the first scholars to call attention to these two parallel developments was Hans-Günter Zmarzlik in his article "Der Sozialdarwinismus in Deutschland als geschichtliches Problem," 253.

4. There is a large secondary literature dealing with Gobineau and his intellectual influence. Some of the more recent works include: George L. Mosse, *Towards the Final Solution*, esp. chap. 4; Michael D. Biddiss, *Father of Racist Theory: The Social and Political Thought of Count Gobineau* (London and New York: Weybright and Talley, 1970); Leon Poliakov, *The Aryan Myth*; Patrik von zur Mühlen, *Rassenideologien*; E. J. Young, *Gobineau und der Rassismus: Eine Kritik der anthropologischen Geschichtstheorie* (Meisenheim am Glan: Anton Hain, 1968); J. R. Baker, *Race* (London: Oxford University Press, 1974).

5. Baker, *Race*, 35.

6. The use of the term *Aryan* as synonymous with "white race" is of course totally incorrect. The word *Aryan* first appears in the early nineteenth century when German philologists sought to lay bare the origins of race by pointing to the common origin of Western languages. The common proto-language was alleged to be Sanskrit, and was said to have been transported from Asia to Europe by the so-called Aryan people. The Aryans were believed to have either originated in or moved into India where they conquered non-Indo-European inhabitants in the area. From here they supposedly migrated to Europe. For a detailed discussion of the tortured history of the term see Mosse, *Toward the Final Solution*, chap. 3.

7. Ibid., 52−54.

8. Ibid., 53.

9. Gobineau used the term "degenerate" in the following manner: "I think that the word 'degenerate' applied to a people should and does signify that this people has no longer the intrinsic value that it formerly possessed, that it no longer has in its veins the same blood, the worth of which has been gradually modified by successive mixtures; or to put it in other words, that with the same name it has not retained the same race as its founder." Quoted in Baker, *Race*, 36.

10. Mühlen, *Rassenideologien*, 67.

11. Mosse, *Toward the Final Solution*, 56.

12. Mühlen, *Rassenideologien*, 116. In France, the term "anthropological sociology" was used to describe the combination of Gobineau's ra-

cism, social Darwinism, and anthropometry. In many ways this term gives a more accurate description of the aims and assumptions of this new discipline than does "social anthropology." In general, it was assumed that there were racial (hence anthropological) differences among various social classes, with the higher social classes exhibiting a higher percentage of Germanic or Nordic stock.

13. For a brief summary of the life and ideas of Lapouge see Eduard Seidler and Günter Nagel, "Georges Vacher de Lapouge (1854–1936) und der Sozialdarwinismus in Frankreich," in *Biologismus im 19. Jahrhundert,* 94–107. See also Clark, *Social Darwinism in France,* 143–154.

14. Poliakov, *The Aryan Myth,* 270.

15. The terms *dolichocephalic* (long-headed) and *brachycephalic* (round-headed) were part of the language of anthropometry (the study of human body measurements) popularized by the École d'Anthropologie. Owing to the belief that the shape of the head was an important criterion of race, in 1840 a process for measuring and differentiating skulls was developed known as the cephalic index. The cephalic index was derived by multiplying the width of the skull by 100 and dividing by the length of the skull. A lower number was characteristic of long-headed dolichocephalic peoples; a higher number indicated an individual was round-headed or brachycephalic. See John Haller, *Outcasts From Evolution: Scientific Attitudes of Racial Inferiority 1859–1900* (Urbana: University of Illinois Press, 1971), esp. chap. 1. In an earlier work, *Les Sélections sociales* (1896), Lapouge called attention to the degeneration of the Aryan race and proposed measures to counteract it.

16. Mühlen, *Rassenideologien,* 90–91; Seidler and Nagel, "de Lapouge," 94–107; Mosse, *Toward the Final Solution,* 58–62. Lapouge's views are best expressed in his two most important works, *L'Aryen, son rôle social* (1899) and *Race et milieu social* (1909). Lapouge sometimes used the word *Aryan* as synonymous with "white race," but seems more frequently to have employed it as equivalent to the so-called Germanic or Nordic race.

17. Otto Ammon's views on the subject can be found in all his works, but are most clearly stated in *Die Gesellschaftsordnung und ihre natürlichen Grundlagen. Entwurf einer Sozial-Anthropologie* (Jena: Gustav Fischer Verlag, 1895), 50–52.

18. Otto Ammon, *Die natürliche Auslese beim Menschen* (Jena: Gustav Fischer Verlag, 1893), 185. Ammon is quoting Lapouge in support of his own position.

19. Ibid., 72.

20. Ibid., 186.

21. For a brief background on the intellectual career of Ludwig Woltmann, see Mosse, *The Crisis of German Ideology* (New York: Grosset and Dunlap, 1964), 99–103.

22. For a discussion of Woltmann's attempt to synthesize socialist, Darwinian, and neo-Kantian thought see Hans-Josef Steinberg, *Sozialismus und deutsche Sozialdemokratie,* 54–55.

23. Mosse, *The Crisis of German Ideology,* 100.

24. Ibid., 100–103.

25. Many of Woltmann's articles appear under pseudonyms; one can only surmise that he hoped thereby to foster the impression that the journal had more regular contributors that it actually enjoyed.

26. Ziegler, "Einleitung zu dem Sammelwerke *Natur und Staat,*" 5.

27. Ibid.

28. For the most part this campaign against Schallmayer and the judges was waged by Woltmann and his colleagues in the *Politisch-anthropologische Revue.* Only Ammon published articles critical of the contest in other journals.

29. Wilhelm Schallmayer, *Beiträge zu einer Nationalbiologie* (Jena: Hermann Costenoble, 1905), 205.

30. Ludwig Woltmann, *Politische Anthropologie* (Leipzig and Eisenach: Eugen, 1903), 1.

31. Ludwig Woltmann, "Nachschrift zu Lapouges Kritik des Jeneser Preisausschreibens," *Politisch-anthropologische Revue* 3 (1904–05): 310.

32. E. Heuppe, Rev. of *Vererbung und Auslese* by W. Schallmayer, *Zeitschrift für Sozialwissenschaft* (1905): 131. Other articles by social anthropologists attacking Schallmayer and the judges include Georges Vacher de Lapouge, "Kritik des Jenenser Preissausschreibens," *Politisch-anthropologische Revue* 3 (1904–05): 297–304; Ludwig Kuhlenbeck, "Kritik der Jenenser Preisschriften," *Politisch-anthropologische Revue* 3 (1904–05): 427–436; Otto Ammon, "Anthropologische Rundschau. Nachwort zum Jenaer sozialanthropologischen Wettbewerb," *Deutsche Welt* (1904): 138–141.

33. Schallmayer, *Beiträge,* 228.

34. Gasman, *Scientific Origins of National Socialism,* 39–40.

35. Schallmayer, *Beiträge,* 203.

36. Ibid., 225.

37. Schallmayer, *Vererbung und Auslese,* 1st ed., 79.

38. Wilhelm Schallmayer, "Gobineaus Rassenwerk und die moderne Gobineauschule," *Zeitschrift für Sozialwissenschaft* 9 (1910): 569–570.

39. Schallmayer, *Vererbung und Auslese,* 2d. ed., 284.

40. Schallmayer, "Gobineaus Rassenwerk," 566.

41. Ibid., 563–564.

42. Ibid., 564.

43. Ibid., 560–561.

44. Wilhelm Schallmayer, "Die soziologische Bedeutung des Nachwuchses der Begabteren und die psychische Vererbung," *ARGB* 2 (1905): 61–63.

45. Schallmayer, *Vererbung und Auslese*, 2d. ed., 38.

46. Schallmayer, "Die soziologische Bedeutung," 63.

47. Schallmayer, "Gobineaus Rassenwerk," 562–563.

48. Schallmayer, *Vererbung und Auslese*, 2d ed., 374.

49. Ibid., 375.

50. Ibid.

51. Schallmayer, "Rassedienst," 435–436.

52. Ibid., 434.

53. Schallmayer, *Vererbung und Auslese*, 2d. ed., 378.

54. Ibid., 376–377.

55. Ibid., 383–384.

56. Ibid., 284.

57. Schallmayer, "Rassedienst," 436.

58. Schallmayer, *Verebung und Auslese*, 2d. ed., 352.

59. Schallmayer's relationship to the Aryan-minded eugenicists will be treated in the Epilogue.

60. My statement that Schallmayer was nonracist holds only for his views regarding the Aryan themes of the Gobineau school. To be sure, Schallmayer did hold racist views with respect to blacks, and to a much lesser degree, Asians—a subject treated in the next chapter. It should be pointed out, however, that even with respect to the latter two groups, his racism was quite moderate compared to most of his contemporaries, especially his fellow eugenicists.

61. By bourgeois social scientists I mean academic social theorists such as Max Weber, Ferdinand Tönnies, and Werner Sombart who, while influenced by Marxism, ultimately rejected the basic tenets of Marx's thought.

62. For a biographical sketch of Ploetz's life see Doeleke, *Alfred Ploetz,* 3–29.

63. The full bibliographical entries are as follows: Alfred Ploetz, "Trostworte an einen naturwissenschaftlichen Hamlet," *ARGB* 29 (1935): 88–89 (reprinted from the *New Yorker Volkszeitung,* Nov. 6, 1892); Ploetz, "Rassentüchtigkeit und Sozialismus," *Neue Deutsche Rundschau* 5 (1894): 989–997; Ploetz, "Sozialpolitik und Rassenhygiene in ihrem prinzipiellen Verhältnis," *Archiv für soziale Gesetzgebung und Statistik* 17

(1902): 393–420; Ploetz, *Tüchtigkeit unsrer Rasse.*

64. Ploetz, "Rassentüchtigkeit," 989–997.

65. Graham, "Science and Values," 1137.

66. Translation of the quotation taken from Graham, "Science and Values," 1137.

67. Ibid.

68. Ploetz, "Sozialpolitik und Rassenhygiene," 393–420.

69. *Verhandlungen des Ersten Deutschen Soziologentages* (Tübingen: J. C. B. Mohr, 1911), 111–165.

70. Ibid., 122.

71. Ibid., 147. This participant, Heinz Potthoff, was a Reichtag deputy. He published a more detailed account of his position in "Schutz der Schwachen," *ARGB* 8 (1911): 86–91.

72. Werner Sombart, "Ideale der Sozialpolitik," *Archiv für soziale Gesetzgebung und Statistik* 10 (1897): 1–48.

73. Ibid., 24–25.

74. Ibid., 8.

75. Ibid., 26–27.

76. *Verhandlungen,* 153.

77. Ibid., 153–154.

78. Ibid., 156–157. I have used the translation from W. G. Runciman, ed., *Weber: Selections in Translation,* trans. Eric Matthews (Cambridge: Cambridge University Press, 1978), 389–390.

79. *Verhandlungen,* 156–157.

80. Schallmayer, *Beiträge,* 154–156.

81. A. Vierkandt, "Ein Einbruch der Naturwissenschaften in die Geisteswissenschaften?" *Zeitschrift für philosophische Kritik* 127 (1906): 170.

82. Ibid., 170–171.

83. A. Vierkandt, "Vererbung und Auslese im Lebenslauf der Völker," *Archiv für die gesamte Psychologie* 7 (1906): 184.

84. Ferdinand Tönnies, "Zur naturwissenschaftlichen Gesellschaftslehre," *Schmollers Jahrbuch für Gesetzgebung und Verwaltung,* 29 (1905): 27–43.

85. Ibid., 44.

86. Schallmayer, *Beiträge,* 209–210.

87. Tönnies wrote an article discussing Galton's views entitled "Eugenik," *Schmollers Jahrbuch für Gesetzgebung und Verwaltung* 29 (1903): 273–290.

88. Tönnies, "Zur naturwissenschaftlichen Gesellschaftslehre," 49–50.

89. Ibid., 53–55.

90. Ibid., 55–56.

91. Ferdinand Tönnies, "Zur naturwissenschaftlichen Gesellschaftslehre. Eine Replik," *Schmollers Jahrbuch für Gestezgebung und Verwaltung* 33 (1907): 94.

92. Ibid.

93. Ibid., 69.

94. Schallmayer, "Einführung in die Rassehygiene," 434.

95. Schallmayer, *Beiträge*, 8.

96. Ibid., 17–18.

97. Ibid., 20–21.

98. Schallmayer, "Soziologische Bedeutung," 38–39.

99. Ibid., 37.

100. Ibid., 40–41.

101. Ibid., 40. Although Sombart claimed that cultural progress was his final goal, hidden behind his rhetoric was the practical aim of preserving the state though economic and social reform. This was the ultimate aim of all the academic social scientists.

102. Schallmayer, *Beiträge*, 32. The biological basis of such asocial activities was, of course, stressed in all his works.

103. John B. Haycraft, *Darwinism and Race Progress* (London: Swan Sonnenschein and Co., 1895). Haycraft is best remembered for his outrageous claim that tuberculosis is a "friend of the race."

104. The contrast between the two traditions was recognized by at least one early twentieth-century hygienist, Dr. W. Oettinger. The introductory remarks of his article "Selektion und Hygiene," *Deutsche Vierteljahrschrift für öffentliche Gesundheitspflege* (1912): 608–626, stimulated my own thought on the subject.

105. German public hygiene, which during most of the nineteenth century had been strictly an empirical and practical branch of medicine lacking its own department in the university, had by 1900 profited from the important discoveries of Robert Koch, Paul Erlich, and others. A more scientific approach to hygiene may be said to have begun when the traditions of Max von Pettenkofer and Robert Koch were combined in the first Prussian chair of hygiene in Göttingen headed by Karl Flügge. For an early twentieth-century appraisal of the development of German hygiene from 1884 to 1909 see Adolf Gottstein, "Die Entwicklung der Hygiene im letzten Vierteljahrhundert," *Zeitschrift für Sozialwissenschaft* 12 (1909): 65–82.

106. For a discussion of the social and political role of hygiene and medicine see chap. 1.

107. Only after the germ theory of disease was firmly established could the link between epidemics and poverty be demonstrated. Gottstein, "Die Entwicklung der Hygiene," 74.

108. See for example Walter Kruse, "Physische Degeneration und Wehrfähigkeit bei europäischen Völkern," *Zentralblatt für allgemeine Gesundheitspflege* 17 (1898): 457–473.

109. Heinrich Herkner, "Die Entartungsfrage in England," *Schmollers Jahrbuch für Gesetzgebung und Verwaltung* 31 (1907): 378.

110. My reason for suggesting a link between the publication of Schallmayer's work and the appearance of the three articles on degeneration is that the hygienists all published their articles in 1903, the year *Vererbung und Auslese* was made available to the public.

111. The articles under discussion are Walter Kruse, "Entartung," *Zeitschrift für Sozialwissenschaft* (1903): 359–376 and 411–434; Friedrich Prinzing, "Die angebliche Wirkung hoher Kindersterblichkeit im Sinne Darwinischer Auslese," *Zentralblatt für allgemeine Gesundheitspflege* (1903): 111–129; Max von Gruber, "Führt die Hygiene zur Entartung der Rasse?" *Münchener medizinische Wochenschrift* 50 (1903): 1713–1718 and 1781–1785.

112. Kruse, "Entartung," 372–374; Prinzing, "Die angebliche Wirkung," 119–121; Gruber, "Führt die Hygiene," 1782.

113. Prinzing, "Die angebliche Wirkung," 111–119, 121–126.

114. Gruber, "Führt die Hygiene," 1715.

115. Kruse, "Entartung," 372.

116. Ibid., 371.

117. Gruber, "Führt die Hygiene," 1782 – 1783.

118. Ibid., 1785.

119. Ibid.

120. Wilhelm Schallmayer, "Wirkungen gebesserter Lebenshaltung und Erfolge der Hygiene als vermeintliche Beweismittel gegen Selektionstheorie und Entartungsfrage," *ARGB* 1 (1904): 54.

121. Ibid., 77.

122. Wilhelm Schallmayer, "Was ist von unserem sozialen Versicherungswesen für die Erbqualitäten der Bevölkerung zu erwarten?" *Archiv für sozialen Hygiene und Demographie* 3 (1909): 61.

123. Wilhelm Schallmayer, "Über das Verhältnis der Individual- und Sozialhygiene zu den Zielen der generativen Hygiene," *Zeitschrift für soziale Medizin* (1906): 337.

124. Schallmayer, "Was ist von unserem sozialen Versicherungswesen," 54.

125. Wihelm Schallmayer, "Kultur und Entartung," *Monatschrift für soziale Medizin und Hygiene* 1 (1906): 482.

126. Schallmayer singled out the eminent social hygienist Alfred Grotjahn as one who neglected this important distinction. Grotjahn tended to use the term degeneration to describe both negative changes in the germ plasma as well as unfavorable acquired conditions, which Schallmayer thought was misleading. Wilhelm Schallmayer, "Sozialhygiene und Eugenik," *Zeitschrift für Sozialwissenschaft* (1914): 397.

127. Schallmayer, "Kultur und Entartung," 483–484.

128. Schallmayer, "Wirkungen gebesserter Lebenshaltung," 76.

129. Schallmayer, "Einführung in die Rassehygiene," 525. Grotjahn was a very active member of the Berlin chapter of the German Society for Race Hygiene. For a brief discussion of his role as physician, social hygienist, and eugenicist see Weindling, "Soziale Hygiene: Eugenik und medizinische Praxis," 6–20.

130. Ibid., 455; Schallmayer, "Sozialhygiene und Eugenik," 330–332.

131. Schallmayer, "Sozialhygiene und Eugenik," 330–332.

132. Schallmayer, "Einführung in die Rassehygiene," 455.

133. Schallmayer, "Sozialhygiene und Eugenik," 331.

134. Schallmayer, "Rassedienst," 439–443.

135. Ibid., 443.

136. Schallmayer, "Sozialhygiene und Eugenik," 331.

137. Ibid., 331–332.

138. Klaus-Dieter Thomann, "Die Zusammenarbeit der Sozialhygieniker Alfred Grotjahn und Alfons Fischer," *Medizinhistorisches Journal* 14 (1979), 252.

139. Otto Peltzer, "Das Verhältnis der Sozialpolitik zur Rassenhygiene: Eine kritische Studie über die Auswirkung biologischer Erkenntnisse auf die Lösungsversuche sozialer Probleme," (Diss., Munich, 1925/26), 39–40.

140. For Schallmayer's discussion of biological policy see *Beiträge*, 63–150.

141. The diagram is a slightly modified version of Schallmayer's own. See Schallmayer, "Einführung in die Rassehygiene," 455.

5: POWER THROUGH POPULATION

1. Schallmayer, *Vererbung und Auslese*, 2d. ed., 353; *Vererbung und Auslese*, 3d. ed., 212–213.

2. Schallmayer, "Zur Bevölkerungspolitik gegenüber dem durch den Krieg verursachten Frauenüberschuß," *ARGB* 11 (1914–15): 729.

3. Hohorst, Kocka, and Ritter, *Sozialgeschichtliches Arbeitsbuch*, 15.

4. Ibid., 29. Demographic historian John Knodel discusses such regional variations, albeit for fertility, not birthrate decline, in his most useful study, *The Decline of Fertility in Germany 1871–1939* (Princeton: Princeton University Press, 1974), 38–69.

5. Hohorst, Kocka, and Ritter, *Sozialgeschichtliches Arbeitsbuch*, 29–30.

6. For a discussion of the number of marriages after 1871 see Knodel, *The Decline of Fertility*, 71. Since infant mortaility was declining, a larger percentage of women reached childbearing age. Ibid., 157.

7. Hohorst, Kocka, and Ritter, *Sozialgeschichtliches Arbeitsbuch*, 29–30; Knodel *The Decline of Fertility*, 96. It should be noted that Knodel's chart reveals statistics on fertility rates, not birthrates; the differences between the two, however, could not have been very significant.

8. Hohorst, Kocka, and Ritter, *Sozialgeschichtliches Arbeitsbuch*, 29–30.

9. Klaus Bade, "German Emigration to the United States and Continental Immigration to Germany in the Late Nineteenth and Early Twentieth Centuries," *Central European History* 13 (1980): 371.

10. Arthur von Fircks, *Bevölkerungslehre und Bevölkerungspolitik*; M. Rubin und H. Westergaard, *Statistik der Ehen auf Grund der sozialen Gliederung der Bevölkerung* (Jena: Gustav Fischer, 1890).

11. Lujo Brentano, "Die Malthusische Lehre und die Bevölkerungsbewegung der letzten Dezennien," *Abhandlungen der Akademie der Wissenschaften* (1908–09): 567–625; Knodel, *The Decline of Fertility*, 127.

12. Julius Wolf, *Der Geburtenrückgang* (Jena: Gustav Fischer, 1912), 42.

13. Ibid.

14. Reinhold Seeberg, *Der Geburtenrückgang in Deutschland* (Leipzig: A. Deichert, 1913), 42–43.

15. German statisticians and eugenicists were constantly pointing to the tremendous decline in France's fertility rate and population growth since the Napoleonic period. They feared, of course, that a similar rapid decline would occur in Germany. See for example Wolf, *Der Geburtenrückgang*, 179, and Schallmayer, *Vererbung und Auslese*, 3d. ed., 217. The fear of depopulation was also an important issue for members of the French eugenics movement. See Schneider, "Toward the Improvement of the Human Race: The History of Eugenics in France," 268–291.

16. To the best of my knowledge, no work exists on Neo-Malthusianism in Germany. Although it probably never possessed as great an institutional base as in England, there must have been some sort of organized activity in Germany, because Schallmayer mentions the existence of a German Neo-Malthusian League (Sozial-harmonischer Verein), which he claims was founded in Stuttgart in 1892. Richard J. Evans in his excellent book, *The Feminist Movement in Germany 1894–1933* (London and Beverly Hills: Sage Publications, 1976) does not discuss

Neo-Malthusianism in detail, and makes no mention of the Sozial-harmonischer Verein. Anything I say regarding Neo-Malthusianism in Germany must hence be tentative; I am unfortunately dependent in large part on Schallmayer's admittedly one-sided appraisal of the movement.

17. For a history of the English Malthusian League see Rosanna Ledbetter, *A History of the Malthusian League 1877–1927* (Columbus: Ohio State University Press, 1976).

18. Richard A. Soloway, "Neo-Malthusians, Eugenists, and the Declining Birth Rate in England, 1900–1918," *Albion* 10 (1978): 272.

19. Ibid., 272–278. Regarding the alleged eugenic effect of birth control, the Neo-Malthusians realized, of course, that the middle classes were employing proportionately far more contraceptives than the working classes, and that this trend was dysgenic. However, as Richard Soloway points out, the Neo-Malthusians believed that contraceptives should be extended to the poor, not taken from the well-to-do. Apparently the Neo-Malthusians, insofar as they concentrated on eugenics, concentrated solely on negative eugenics.

20. Evans, *The Feminist Movement*, 9–23.

21. The percentage of women white-collar workers climbed from 3.7 percent in 1882 to 12.4 percent in 1907. Hohorst, Kocka, and Ritter, *Sozialgeschichtliches Arbeitsbuch*, 67.

22. Evans, *The Feminist Movement*, 17–20.

23. Ibid., 20–22.

24. Ibid., 37.

25. Ibid., 1.

26. Ibid., 131.

27. For a discussion of the so-called new morality, see Evans, *The Feminist Movement*, 115–143.

28. Ibid., 131.

29. Ibid., 132.

30. For a discussion of the Mutterschutz League see Evans, *The Feminist Movement*, 115–143.

31. The term *gelbe Gefahr* (yellow peril) was coined by Emperor William II at the time of the Boxer Rebellion in China. It became especially popular after the Japanese victory in the Russo-Japanese War of 1904–1905. Geoffrey Barraclough, *An Introduction to Contemporary History* (New York: Penguin, 1981), 81.

32. Ibid., 80.

33. As one German author explained in his popular book written shortly after the Boxer Rebellion, China, owing to its formidable intellectual tradition and moral system as well as its colossal population, was potentially more dangerous than Japan. Hermann von Samson-

Himmelstjerna, *Die gelbe Gefahr als Moralproblem* (Berlin: Deutscher Kolonial Verlag, 1902).

34. Schallmayer, *Vererbung und Auslese,* 3d. ed., 218–219.

35. Volker R. Berghahn, *Germany and the Approach of War in 1914* (London: Macmillan Press, 1973), 47, 51, 63, 77, 80, 131, 137, 157, 167, and 169; Schallmayer, "Die Politik der Fruchtbarkeitsbeschränkungen," *Zeitschrift für Politik* 2 (1908): 411.

36. Concerning this point see, for example, Karl von Behr-Pinnow, *Geburtenrückgang und Bekämpfung der Sauglingsterblichkeit* (Berlin: J. Springer, 1913), 37. On the question of the danger of the two-child system, Julius Wolf, quoting eugenics supporter Pontus Fahlbeck, had the following to say: "especially in a time of general intellectual uncertainty, like the present, and for a nation with dangerous neighbors, the [two-child] system is the sure way to a fast decline." Wolf, *Der Geburtenrückgang,* 186.

37. Schallmayer, *Vererbung und Auslese,* 3d ed., 194.

38. Ibid., 195.

39. Ibid., 201–202.

40. Ibid., 202.

41. Ibid.

42. Ibid.

43. Ibid., 205.

44. Ibid., 206.

45. Ibid., 211.

46. Schallmayer, "Die Politik der Fruchtbarkeitsbeschränkungen," 393.

47. Schallmayer, rev. of *Rassenverbesserung, Malthusianismus und Neumalthusianismus,* by Johannes Rutgers, *ARGB* 5 (1908): 827.

48. For a discussion of eugenically minded Neo-Malthusianism in England see Soloway, "Neo-Malthusians," 264–286.

49. Schallmayer, rev. of *Rassenverbesserung, Malthusianismus und Neumalthusianismus,* by Johannes Rutgers, 831.

50. Ibid., 832.

51. Ibid.

52. Ibid., 833.

53. The term *maternal selection* was not used by Rutgers as such, although it accurately reflects his views. Rutgers expected that women, by deciding whether or not to have children, would in effect be taking selection into their own hands; he described the use of contraceptives by females for purposes of family planning as "Auslese durch die Mutter." Johannes Rutgers, *Rassenverbesserung, Malthusianismus und Neumalthusianismus,* trans. Martina G. Kramers (Dresden and Leipzig: Heinrich Minden, 1908), 229.

54. Schallmayer, rev. of *Rassenverbesserung, Malthusianismus und Neumalthusianismus,* by Johannes Rutgers, 834.

55. Schallmayer, "Eugenik, ihre Grundlagen und ihre Beziehungen zur kulturellen Hebung der Frau," *Archiv für Frauenkunde und Konstitutiônsforschung* (1914): 288.

56. Ibid.

57. Sebald R. Steinmetz, "Feminismus und Rasse," *Zeitschrift für Sozialwissenschaft* 7 (1904): 758.

58. Schallmayer, "Eugenik," 289.

59. Ibid.

60. For an excellent discussion of the relationship between declining fertility and the cult of motherhood in England see Anna Davin, "Imperialism and Motherhood," *History Workshop,* no. 5 (1978): 9–65; Schallmayer, *Vererbung und Auslese,* 3d ed., 332.

61. Schallmayer, "Eugenik," 290.

62. Pamphlet "Was will die Deutsche Gesellschaft für Bevölkerungspolitik" in Bundesarchiv Koblenz, R 86, 2371, Bd. II, fol. 117–118. Although no exact date appears on the document, from its position in the document bundle, it was probably published in the early part of 1919. From a 1915 report by Lenz discussing the aims of the Society, it is clear that its objectives were not different before the war. See Fritz Lenz, "Deutsche Gesellschaft für Bevölkerungspolitik," *ARGB* 11 (1914–1915): 555–557.

63. Ibid., 556. It is obvious from the strong nationalistic and overly defensive tone of the society's proclamation (*Propaganda-Aufruf*) that the society owed its formation to the then all-pervasive wartime paranoia regarding population decline.

64. Ibid., 554–557; Schallmayer, "Neue Aufgaben und neue Organisation der Gesundheitspolitik," *Archiv für soziale Hygiene und Demographie* 13 (1919): 258–259.

65. The only pieces of evidence known to the author which suggest that the government was at least aware of, if not overly concerned about, eugenics prior to the war are two memos sent to German Chancellor von Bülow from the German consulate in Washington, D.C. sometime between 1900 and 1909. Unfortunately the documents were not dated. The first memo contains a report on the Michigan eugenics-related sterilization law; the second includes a report on marriage procedures in the United States. Bundesarchiv Koblenz, R 86, 2371, Bd. I, fol. 18 and 19.

66. Schallmayer, "Bevölkerungspolitische Kriegsliteratur," *Zeitschrift für Politik* 10 (1917): 441. Both Schallmayer and Lenz give a detailed report of the October meeting and the issues discussed there. Ibid., 441–459; Fritz Lenz, "Notizen," *ARGB* 12 (1916–1918): 116–124. A compilation of the views of the numerous participants are recorded in a 291-

page pamphlet entitled, *Die Erhaltung und Vermehrung der deutschen Volkskraft. Verhandlungen der 8. Konferenz der Zentralstelle für Volkswohlfahrt in Berlin vom 26. bis 28. Oktober 1915* (Berlin: Heymann, 1916); Schallmayer, "Bevölkerungspolitische," 460.

67. Schallmayer, "Zur Bevölkerungspolitik," 729.

68. Schallmayer, "Kriegswirkungen am Volkskörper und ihre Heilung," *Die Umschau* 22 (1918): 22. Schallmayer did not expect the revolution and subsequent new order in Russia to alter the country's imperialist and expansionist designs. "Die augenblickliche Vorherrschaft demokratischer Grundsätze in Russland gibt us noch lange keine Sicherheit gegen das Wiederaufkommen des russischen Imperialismus mit seiner jahrhundertlang unablässig geübten Expansionstendenz, die nicht nur für uns und unsere Verbündeten, sondern, was merkwürdig selten bedacht wird, auch für das übrige Europa eine rechternstliche Gefahr bedeutet." Schallmayer expected Russia to withstand population losses better than Germany because of its high fertility rate, and its potentially large decrease in the country's mortality rate.

69. Ibid., 1. Schallmayer was so concerned about the issue of "excess of women" following the war that he devoted an entire article to it. See Schallmayer, "Zur Bevölkerungspolitik," 713–737.

70. Schallmayer, "Kriegswirkungen," 3.

71. Schallmayer, "Zur Bevölkerungspolitik," 714.

72. For a discussion of all his proposals see Schallmayer, *Vererbung und Auslese*, 3d ed., 325–367.

73. Ibid., 336.

74. Ibid., 339.

75. Ibid., 351.

76. Lenz, "Rassenhygienische Bevölkerungspolitik," *Deutsche Politik* 1 (1916): 1665.

77. Schallmayer, *Vererbung und Auslese*, 3d ed., 352.

78. For an example of Lenz's nationalist views and his fear of the Russians see Lenz, "Vorschläge zur Bevölkerungspolitik mit besonderer Berücksichtigung der Wirtschaftslage nach dem Krieg," *ARGB* 12 (1916–1918): 445.

79. Schallmayer, *Vererbung und Auslese*, 3d ed., 352.

80. Ibid., 339–344; 344–350; 357–360.

81. These ten "guiding principles" formulated by the Delegate Committee of the German Society for Race Hygiene in June, 1914 are listed in Schallmayer's text. Schallmayer, *Vererbung und Auslese*, 3d ed., 359–360.

82. Lenz, "Rassenhygienische Bevölkerungspolitik," 1668.

83. Since Schallmayer never made any direct statements concerning the political situation after the war, this must remain somewhat specula-

tive. I have been unable to detect any change of intellectual orientation in the three articles he wrote after the war. My impression from reading these articles is that he moved neither to the left nor to the right politically. Regarding socialism and, by extension, the new social democratic order in Germany, he stated that he "expected neither more nor less now than he did over the past decades." Schallmayer, "Der Sozialismus vom gesellschaftsbiologischen Standpunkt," *Die Umschau* 23 (1919): 18.

84. Schallmayer reaffirmed this view in an article written during the last year of his life. Schallmayer, "Der Sozialismus," 17–20.

EPILOGUE

1. Hermann Siemens, *Die biologischen Grundlagen*, 10–11.

2. Max von Gruber, "Wilhelm Schallmayer," *ARGB* 14 (1922): 52.

3. Fritz Lenz, "Wilhelm Schallmayer," *Münchener medizinische Wochenschrift* 66 (1919): 1294–1296.

4. This point is discussed in two letters from Wilhelm Schallmayer to the Swiss eugenicist August Forel. The first dates from April 24, 1906. See Hans Walser, ed., *August Forel. Briefe—Correspondenz 1864–1927* (Bern: Hans Huber, 1968), 383. The second was found in the August Forel Archive of the University of Zürich and was kindly brought to my attention by Dr. Peter Zörner. Its date is illegible.

5. See for example Fritz Lenz's justification of the term *Rassenhygiene* in Lenz, "Zum Begriff der Rassenhygiene und seine Benennung," *ARGB* 11 (1914–15): 445–448.

6. Ploetz, "Unser Weg" (pamphlet found in the Ploetz family archive), 2.

7. *Widar-Blätter*, no. 1 (August 1919): 1–10.

8. Alfred Ploetz, "Ziele und Aufgabe der Rassenhygiene," *Vierteljahrsschrift für öffentliche Gesundheitspflege* 43 (1911): 190; Erwin Baur, Eugen Fischer, and Fritz Lenz, *Grundriß der menschlichen Erblichkeitslehre und Rassenhygiene* (Munich: J. F. Lehmann, 1923), 2:206.

9. The name "German Society for Race Hygiene" dates only as far back as 1910. Between 1905 and 1907 the society appears to have simply been called Gesellschaft für Rassenhygiene. From 1907 to 1910 the society was known as the Internationale Gesellschaft für Rassenhygiene— reflecting Ploetz's hope that the Society would attract a large number of foreign members. When it became clear that non-German eugenicists were more inclined to join eugenics organizations in their own countries, Ploetz and other German eugenicists officially changed the name

of the society. The criteria for membership discussed in the text refer to those of the 1905–1907 society. Alfred Ploetz, "2. Bericht der Internationalen Gesellschaft für Rassenhygiene" (report found in the Ploetz family archive), 3.

10. Gruber, "Wilhelm Schallmayer," 55.

11. Georg Lilienthal has suggested that the society actually split. Lilienthal, "Rassenhygiene im Dritten Reich," 117; Paul Weindling rightly points out the serious tensions between the Berlin and Munich chapters of the society, but does not suggest that there were two movements. Weindling, "Weimar Eugenics," 315. For a discussion of these tensions between nonracist and racist eugenicists during the Weimar period see my forthcoming article, "The Race Hygiene Movement in Germany," in *Osiris* 3 (1987).

12. Emphasis in the original. Form letter by E. Baur et al., for the Berliner Gesellschaft für Rassenhygiene, 18 Dec. 1917, Bundesarchiv, R86, 2371, fol. 90.

13. "Geleitwort," *Eugenik* 1 (1930): n.p.

14. *Eugenik* was the successor journal to the Berlin *Volksaufartung, Erblehre, Eheberatung* (1928–1930), which in turn succeeded the *Zeitschrift für Volksaufartung und Erbkunde* (1926–1927). Unlike its predecessors, however, *Eugenik* was not officially tied to the Deutscher Bund für Volksaufartung (German Alliance for National Regeneration), a nonracist Berlin-based organization comprised primarily of eugenically-minded Prussian civil servants. It had a more left-wing and populist orientation than the society and eventually merged with the latter in 1931.

15. Hermann Muckermann, "Illustrationen zu der Frage: Wohlfahrtspflege und Eugenik," *Eugenik* 2 (1931): 42.

16. "Eugenische Tagung des Preussischen Landesgesundheitsrates," *Eugenik* 2 (1931–1932): 187–189; Lilienthal, "Rassenhygiene im Dritten Reich," 119–120; Joachim Müller, "Sterilisation und Gestzgebung bis 1933" (paper delivered at the Institute for the History of Medicine in Mainz, 7 Nov. 1978), 13–18. Although under the 1932 proposal sterilization would have remained *legally* voluntary—and this is an important difference between it and the Nazi Law—it was hardly "voluntary" in the sense that those who were to undergo the operation could make a free choice. Termination of welfare support was just one of the many indirect coercive methods used to ensure the prospective candidates' compliance. It goes without saying that none of the German eugenicists viewed sterilization as a "right" that individuals could exercise to satisfy their own personal needs; it was a technology to be employed in the service of the "health of the nation." Bock, Gisela, *Zwangssterilisation im Nationalsozialismus*, 49–52.

17. Bock, *Zwangssterilisation im Nationalsozialismus*, 80. For a discussion of the requests for sterilization see 80–83.

18. Lilienthal, "Rassenhygiene im Dritten Reich," 120.

19. Lenz, "Die Stellung des Nationalsozialismus zur Rassenhygiene," *ARGB* 25 (1931): 300.

20. Lenz found Hitler's rabid anti-Semitism too extreme. Ibid., 302.

21. Ibid., 301.

22. On May 26, 1933, several months prior to the sterilization law of July, 1933, eugenic sterilizations were effectively legalized by changing the wording of an already existing law dealing with "bodily injury." Although it did not mention the word "eugenic," the new addition to §226 (§226a) was designed to enable physicians to sterilize "defective" individuals without fear of prosecution. Under §226a patients (or their legal guardians) were still required to give their consent to the operation. However, the voluntary nature of this "consent" must be called into question when one considers that it was often presented to patients as a condition for their release from an asylum. Bock, *Zwangssterilisation im Nationalsozialismus*, 83.

23. "Gesetz zur Verhütung erbkranken Nachwuchses," *ARGB* 27 (1933): 420–423; Robert N. Proctor, "Pawns or Pioneers? The Role of Doctors in the Origins of Nazi Racial Science" (Ms, Harvard University, 1982), 44.

24. Bock, *Zwangssterilisation im Nationalsozialismus*, 84. The proposal was probably drafted by the Director of the Commission of National Health Service, Dr. Arthur Gütt. Proctor, "Pawns or Pioneers," 45.

25. Bock, *Zwangssterilisation im Nationalsozialismus*, 85.

26. Baader and Schultz, *Medizin und Nationalsozialismus*, 145–146. The estimated cost for sterilizing the "defective" and the estimated financial savings was reported in a letter to the *Journal of the American Medical Association* 102 (1934): 630–631. See William E. Seidelmann, "From Hippocrates to the Holocaust," unpub. paper delivered at McMaster University, Hamilton, Ontario, Canada, February 14, 1985, 7.

27. Bock, *Zwangssterilisation im Nationalsozialismus*, 237–238; Gisela Bock, "Racism and Sexism in Nazi Germany: Motherhood, Compulsory Sterilization, and the State," in *When Biology Became Destiny: Women in Weimar and Nazi Germany*, ed. Renate Bridenthal, Atina Grossmann, and Marion Kaplan (New York: Monthly Review Press, 1984), 279–280. According to Bock, approximately 53% were sterilized for "feeblemindedness" and about 20% for "schizophrenia." Between 1934 and 1937, approximately 80 men and 400 women died as a result of the operation.

28. Bock, "Racism and Sexism in Nazi Germany," 280–282.

29. Proctor, "Pawns or Pioneers," 78.

30. Bock, *Zwangssterilisation im Nationalsozialismus*, 94–95. The 1935

revision of the sterilization law allowed for the castration of homosexuals with their "consent."

31. For a brief discussion of these pronatal strategies see Bock, "Racism and Sexism in Nazi Germany," 276–277; a far more exhaustive treatment can be found in Bock's book. One of Bock's most valuable contributions is her demonstration that, contrary to popular belief, antinatalism rather than pronatalism was the more significant feature of Nazi racial and population policy. The two, however, went hand in hand. It should, of course, be noted that there were also explicitly racist pronatal policies. The best example of this was Himmler's *Lebensborn* program. For a full account of its history see Lilienthal, *Der "Lebensborn e. V."*

32. Bock, "Racism and Sexism," 277.

33. At this time the society came under the "Führer principle," which meant loss of any independence and democratic control.

34. Richard Goldschmidt held a post in the prestigious Kaiser-Wilhelm Institut für Biologie in Berlin until he, like most Jewish civil servants, was dismissed from his post with the passage of the Law for the Restoration of the Professional Civil Service on April 7, 1933. Goldschmidt was a strong advocate of sterilization legislation during the late Weimar years. Weindling, "Weimar Eugenics," 309, 315.

35. Lilienthal, "Rassenhygiene im Dritten Reich," 123.

36. See, for example, Otto Helmut, *Volk in Gefahr: Der Geburtenrückgang und seine Folgen für Deutschlands Zukunft* (Munich: J. F. Lehmann, 1934) and Friedrich Burgdörfer, *Völker am Abgrund* (Munich: J. F. Lehmann, 1936).

37. The terms Erbpflege and Rassenpflege are discussed in Otto Freiherr von Verschuer, *Leitfaden der Rassenhygiene* (Leipzig: Georg Thieme, 1941), 125; and in an article by Arthur Gütt, "Auslese und Lebensauslese in ihre Bedeutung für Erbgesundheit und Rassenpflege," in *Erblehre und Rassenhygiene im völkischen Staat,* ed. Ernst Rüdin (Munich: J. F. Lehmann, 1934), 118.

38. It should be noted that with possible exception of Lenz, who served on a committee designed to formulate a law permitting euthanasia—a law that never saw the light of day because the action always remained officially secret—the professional eugenicists were not involved in this incident directly, and did not view it as a part of race hygiene. Indeed, according to Weindling, Rüdin apparently suffered a loss of funds owing to his refusal to go along with euthanasia. Weindling, "Race, Blood, and Politics," 13. This does not mean, of course, that the action was not known and at least half-heartedly supported by

many active race hygienists. There is an extensive literature on this tragic episode. The most exhaustive account is Ernst Klee, *"Euthanasie" im NS-Staat. Die "Vernichtung lebensunwerten Lebens"* (Frankfurt am Main: S. Fischer, 1983). Other accounts include Benno Müller-Hill, *Tödliche Wissenschaft;* Kurt Nowak, *"Euthanasie" und Sterilisierung im Dritten Reich. Die Konfrontation der evangelischen und katholischen Kirche mit dem "Gesetz zur Verhütung erbkranken Nachwuchses" und der "Euthanasie"-Aktion,* 3d ed. (Göttingen: Vandenhoeck und Ruprecht, 1984); Baader and Schultz, *Medizin und Nationalsozialismus,* 95–101; Proctor, "Pawns or Pioneers," 93–102; Frederic Wertham, *A Sign for Cain* (New York: Werner Paperback Library, 1973), chapter 9; Alice Platen-Hallermond, *Die Tötung Geisteskranken in Deutschland* (Frankfurt am Main: Frankfurter Hefte, 1948); Alexander Mitschelich and Fred Mielke, eds., *Medizin ohne Menschlichkeit: Dokumente des Nürnberger Ärzteprozesses* (Frankfurt am Main: S. Fischer, 1978); Klaus Dörner, "Nationalsozialismus und Lebensvernichtung," *Vierteljahrshefte für Zeitgeschichte* 15 (1967): 121–152; Karl Heinz Hafner and Rolf Winau, "'Die Freigabe der Vernichtung lebensunwerten Lebens': Eine Untersuchung zu der Schrift von Karl Binding und Alfred Hoche," *Medizinhistorisches Journal* 9 (1974): 227–254.

39. Most provocative in the elaboration of this view is Richard L. Rubenstein's *The Cunning of History: The Holocaust and the American Future* (New York: Harper & Row, 1975), 33. Rubenstein argues that Germany's Jews became "surplus people" through a bureaucratic sleight-of-hand: the removal of their citizenship in 1935. Once most of Europe's Jews became stateless and rightless, argues Rubenstein, the Nazis violated no law by exterminating them since these people were no longer covered by any law.

40. Müller-Hill, *Tödliche Wissenschaft,* 73–74. The connection of "eugenic racism" and "bureaucratic, scientific and faultlessly efficient genocide of the scale of the Holocaust" is also advanced by Gisela Bock in "Racism and Sexism in Nazi Germany," 283, although my own views were arrived at without prior knowledge of her outstanding work.

BIBLIOGRAPHY

A NOTE ON ARCHIVAL SOURCES

Schallmayer's personal papers, which had been housed at the former Race Hygiene Institute in Jena, appear to have been completely destroyed in the closing days of World War II. A few scattered letters exist in various collections, such as the letters to Forel which are located in the Forel papers at the University of Zürich. Some letters to Ploetz, as well as a large collection of completely unsorted material on the German eugenics movement, exist in the private archive of the Ploetz family in Herrsching, West Germany. I have been told of the existence of several letters to Alfred Grotjahn in the Grotjahn papers at the Humboldt University in Berlin, German Democratic Republic. A few scattered pieces of information on the Krupp competition can be found in the Ernst-Haeckel-Haus in Jena, GDR (Best. A-Abt. 1 No n 0005) and in the Krupp Archive, Essen, West Germany (IX d 244 and III d 159). At the Bundesarchiv Koblenz (West German Federal Archive) there is relatively little material on eugenics in the Wilhelmine period (see R 86, 2371, Bd. I-II). Overall the archival material existing for Schallmayer is insufficient for an in-depth biographical portrait.

INTERVIEWS

Ploetz, Wilfrid. Interview with author. Herrsching, West Germany, 1978.
Schallmayer, Friedrich. Interview with author. Karlsruhe, West Germany,
1977, 1984.

SCHALLMAYER'S PUBLICATIONS

"Auslese beim Menschen: Eine Erwiderung." *Zeitschrift für philosophische Kritik* 129 (1907): 136–154.

"Die Auslesewirkungen des Krieges." *Menschheitsziele* (1908):381–385.

"Eine Ausschau für die Friedensfreunde." *Das neue Jahrhundert* 2
(1899):771–773, 788–791.

Beiträge zu einer Nationalbiologie. Jena: Hermann Costenoble, 1905.

"Zur Bevölkerungspolitik gegenüber dem durch den Krieg verursachten
Frauenüberschuss." *ARGB* 11 (1914–1915):713–737.

"Bevölkerungspolitische Kriegsliteratur." *Zeitschrift für Politik* 10
(1917):441–468.

"Brauchen wir eine Rassehygiene?" *Der praktische Arzt* (1916): 47–50,
71–74, 170–176, 195–202.

*Die drohende physische Entartung der Culturvölker und die Verstaatlichung
des ärztlichen Standes.* 2d ed. Berlin and Neuwied: Heuser, 1895.

"Zum Einbruch der Naturwissenschaften in das Gebiet der
Geisteswissenschaften." *ARGB* 1 (1904):586–597.

"Einführung in die Rassehygiene." In *Ergebnisse der Hygiene, Bakteriologie, Immunitätsforschung und experimentalen Therapie,* edited by
W. Weichards, 2:433–532. Berlin: J. Springer, 1917.

"Die Erbentwicklung bei Völkern als theoretisches und praktisches
Problem." *Menschheitsziele* (1907):44–49, 92–97.

"Ernst Haeckel und die Eugenik." In *Was Wir Ernst Haeckel Verdanken,*
edited by Heinrich Schmidt, 2:367–372. Leipzig: Unesma, 1914.

"Eugenik, ihre Grundlagen und ihre Beziehungen zur kulturellen
Hebung der Frau." *Archiv für Frauenkunde und Konstitutionsforschung*
(1914):281–291.

"Eugenik, Lebenshaltung und Auslese." *Zeitschrift für Sozialwissenschaft*
11 (1908):267–277.

"Frauenfortschritt und Volksnachwuchs." *Das kommende Geschlecht* 1
(1921):17–21.

"Generative Ethik." *ARGB* 6 (1909):199–231.

"Gobineaus Rassenwerk und die moderne Gobineauschule." *Zeitschrift für Sozialwissenschaft,* N.F., 1 (1910):553–572.

"Grundlinien der Vererbungslehre." In *Künstliche Fehlgeburt und künstliche Unfruchtbarkeit: Ihre Indikationen, Technik und Rechtslage,* edited by Siegfried Placzek, 1–48. Leipzig: G. Thieme, 1918.

"Infektion als Morgengabe." *Zeitschrift für Bekämpfung der Geschlechtskrankheiten* 2 (1903–1904):389–419.

"Der Krieg als Züchter." *ARGB* 5 (1908):364–400.

"Kriegswirkungen am Volkskörper und ihre Heilung." *Die Umschau* 22 (1918):1–24.

"Kultur und Entartung." *Monatsschrift für soziale Medizin und Hygiene* 1 (1906):481–495, 544–554.

"Ein Medizinalministerium." *Das neue Jahrhundert* 2 (1899):390–395.

"Die Nahrungsverweigerung und die übrigen Störungen der Nahrungsaufnahme bei Geisteskranken." Med. diss., Munich, 1885.

"Natürliche und geschichtliche Auslese bei wilden und bei hochkultivierten Völkern." *Politisch-anthropologische Revue* 1 (1902): 245–272.

"Neue Aufgaben und neue Organisation der Gesundheitspolitik." *Archiv für Hygiene und Demographie* 13 (1919):225–270.

"Die Politik der Fruchtbarkeitsbeschränkungen." *Zeitschrift für Politik* 2 (1908):391–439.

"Rassedienst." *Sexualprobleme* (1911):433–443, 534–547.

"Rassehygiene und sonstige Hygiene." *ARGB* 9 (1912):217–221.

"Rassehygiene und Sozialismus." *Die neue Zeit* 25 (1906–1907):731–740.

"Rasseprobleme." *Zeitschrift für Politik* 8 (1914):412–427.

Review of *Rassenverbesserung, Malthusianismus und Neumalthusianismus,* by Johannes Rutgers. *ARGB* 5 (1908):826–835.

"Selektive Gesichtspunkte zur generativen und kulturellen Völkerentwicklung." *Schmollers Jahrbuch für Gesetzgebung und Verwaltung* 30 (1906):421–449.

"Sicherung des Volksnachwuchses und Sozialisierung der Nachwuchskosten." *Die Umschau* 23 (1919):497–500, 517–520.

"Soziale Maßnahmen zur Verbesserung der Fortpflanzungsauslese." In *Krankheit und soziale Lage,* edited by M. Mosse and G. Tugendreich, 841–859. Munich: J. F. Lehmann, 1913.

"Sozialhygiene und Eugenik." *Zeitschrift für Sozialwissenschaft,* N. F., 5 (1914):329–339, 397–408, 505–513.

"Der Sozialismus vom gesellschaftsbiologischen Standpunkt." *Die Umschau* 23 (1919):17–20.

"Sozialistische Entwicklungs- und Bevölkerungslehre." *Zeitschrift für Sozialwissenschaft,* N. F., 2 (1911):511–530.

"Die soziologische Bedeutung des Nachwuchses der Begabteren und die psychische Vererbung." *ARGB* 2 (1905):36–75.

"Über das Verhältnis der Individual- und Sozialhygiene zu den Zielen der generativen Hygiene." *Zeitschrift für soziale Medizin* 2 (1906):331–343.

"Über die Grundbedeutung der Ethik und ihr Verhältnis zu den Forderungen des Rassedienstes." *Die neue Generation* 6 (1910):433–438, 483–496.

"Unzeitgemässe Gedanken über Europas Zukunft." *ARGB* 11 (1914–1915):449–456.

Vererbung und Auslese als Faktoren zur Tüchtigkeit und Entartung der Völker. Flugschriften des deutschen Monistenbundes, no. 5. Brackweide i. W.: W. Breitenbach, 1907.

Vererbung und Auslese im Lebenslauf der Völker: Eine staatswissenschaftliche Studie auf Grund der neueren Biologie. 1st ed. Jena: Gustav Fischer, 1903.

Vererbung und Auslese in ihrer soziologischen und politischen Bedeutung. 2d ed. Jena: Gustav Fischer, 1910.

Vererbung und Auslese: Grundriss der Gesellschaftsbiologie und der Lehre vom Rassedienst. 3d ed. Jena: Gustav Fischer, 1918.

"Was ist von unserem sozialen Versicherungswesen für die Erbqualitäten der Bevölkerung zu erwarten?" *Archiv für sozialen Hygiene und Demographie* 3 (1909):27–65.

"Wirkungen gebesserter Lebenshaltung und Erfolge der Hygiene als vermeintliche Beweismittel gegen Selektionstheorie und Entartungsfrage." *ARGB* 1 (1904):53–77.

PUBLICATIONS BEFORE 1945

Ackerknecht, Erwin H. "Beiträge zur Geschichte der Medizinalreform von 1848." *Sudhoffs Archiv für Geschichte der Medizin* 25 (1932):61–183.

Alsberg, Moritz. "Erbliche Entartung bedingt durch soziale Einflüsse." *Frankfurter Zeitung,* Sept. 24, 1903.

———. *Erbliche Entartung bedingt durch soziale Einflüsse.* Kassel and Leipzig: T. G. Fischer, 1903.

Ammon, Otto. *Die Gesellschaftsordnung und ihre natürlichen Grundlagen.* Jena: Gustav Fischer, 1895.

———. "Nachwort zum Jenaer sozialanthropologischen Wettbewerb." *Deutsche Welt* (1904):138–141.

———. *Die natürliche Auslese beim Menschen.* Jena: Gustav Fischer, 1893.

———. Rev. of *Vererbung und Auslese,* by W. Schallmayer. *Deutsche Welt* (1903):172–174.

———. Rev. of *Vererbung und Auslese,* by W. Schallmayer. *Naturwissenschaftliche Wochenschrift* (1904):221–223.

Arndt, Rudolf. *Die Neurasthenie (Nervenschwäche). Ihr Wesen, Ihre Bedeutung und Behandlung.* Vienna and Leipzig: Urban Schwarzenberg, 1885.

Aronsohn, Oscar. *Ueber Heredität bei Epilepsie.* Berlin: Wilhelm Axt, 1894.

Aschaffenburg, Gustav. *Crime and Its Repression.* Trans. Adalbert Albrecht. Boston: Little, Brown and Co., 1913.

Baur, Erwin. *Einführung in die experimentelle Vererbungslehre.* Berlin: Gebrüder Borntraeger, 1911.

Baur, Erwin, Fischer, Eugen, and Lenz, Fritz. *Menschliche Erblichkeitslehre und Rassenhygiene.* 2d ed. Munich: J. F. Lehmann, 1923.

———. *Grundriß der menschlichen Erblichkeitslehre und Rassenhygiene.* 2 vols. 4th ed. Munich: J. F. Lehmann, 1936(vol. 1), 1932 (vol. 2).

Beard, George. *American Nervousness: Its Causes and Consequences.* New York: G. P. Putnam's Sons, 1881.

Bebel, August. *Die Frau und der Sozialismus.* 1909. Reprint. Frankfurt am Main: Marxistische Blätter, 1977.

Behr-Pinnow, Karl von. *Geburtenrückgang und Bekämpfung der Sauglingssterblichkeit.* Berlin: J. Springer, 1913.

Bernstein, Eduard. "Ludwig Woltmanns Beziehungen zur Sozialdemokratie." *Politisch-anthropologische Revue* 6 (1907–1908):45–53.

Biermann, E. "Sozialwissenschaft, Geschichte und Naturwissenschaft." *Conrads Jahrbücher für Nationalökonomie* 28 (1904):592–607.

Binswanger, Otto. "Geistesstörung und Verbrechen." *Deutsche Rundschau* 57 (1888):419–440.

———. *Die Pathologie und Therapie der Neurasthenie. Vorlesungen für Studierende und Aerzte.* Jena: Gustav Fischer, 1896.

Blaschko, Alfred. "Bemerkungen zur Weismann'schen Theorie." *Die neue Zeit* 13 (1894–1895):119–122.

——. *Geburtenrückgang und Geschlechtskrankheiten.* Leipzig: Johann Ambrosius Barth, 1914.

——. "Hygiene der Prostitution und venerische Krankheiten." In *Handbuch der Hygiene.* Ed. T. Weyl, vol. 2. Jena: Gustav Fischer, 1901.

——. "Natürliche Auslese und Klassenteilung." *Die neue Zeit* 13 (1894–1895):615–624.

Bleuler, E. "Führen die Fortschritte der Medizin zur Entartung der Rasse." *Münchener medizinische Wochenschrift* 51 (1904):312–313.

Bluhm, Agnes. "Rassenhygiene." *Concordia: Zeitschrift der Centralstelle für Arbeiterwohlfahrtseinrichtungen* 24 (1917):287.

——. "Die soziale Versicherung im Lichte der Rassenhygiene." *ARGB* 12 (1916–1918):15–42.

——. "Die Stillungsnot, ihre Ursachen und die Vorschläge zu ihrer Bekämpfung." *Zeitschrift für soziale Medizin* 3 (1907–1908):72–78, 160–172, 261–270, 357–387.

——. "Zur Frage nach der generativen Tüchtigkeit der deutschen Frauen und der rassenhygienischen Bedeutung der ärztlichen Geburtshilfe." *ARGB* 9 (1912):330–346, 454–474.

Bollinger, O. "Ueber Vererbung von Krankheiten." In *Beiträge zur Biologie als Festgabe dem Anatomen und Physiologen. Th. von Bischoff zum fünfzigjährigen medizinischen Doktorjubiläum gewidmet von seinen Schülern,* 271–294. Stuttgart: J. G. Cotta, 1882.

Boring, Edwin G. *A History of Experimental Psychology.* New York and London: D. Appleton and Co., 1929.

Bornträger, Jean. *Der Geburtenrückgang in Deutschland: Seine Bewertung und Bekämpfung.* Würzburg: Curt Kabitzsch, 1913.

Braencker, Wilhelm. *Die Entstehung der Eugenik in England.* Hildburghausen: L. Nonnes, 1917.

Brentano, Lujo. "Die Malthusische Lehre und die Bevölkerungsbewegung der letzten Dezennien." *Abhandlungen der Akademie der Wissenschaften* (1908–1909):567–625.

Buchner, H. Rev. of *Über die drohende körperliche Entartung der Kulturmenscheit,* by W. Schallmayer. *Münchener medizinische Wochenschrift* (1892):478–480.

Bumke, Oswald. *Über nervöse Entartung.* Berlin: J. Springer, 1912.

Damm, Alfred. *Die Entartung der Menschen und die Beseitigung der Entartung.* Berlin: Bruer, 1895.

Daniels, E. Rev. of *Vererbung und Auslese,* by W. Schallmayer. *Preussische Jahrbücher* (1904):342–347.

Darwin, Charles. *Descent of Man and Selection in Relation to Sex.* 2d ed. 1876. Reprint. New York: The Modern Library, n.d.

————. *The Variation of Animals and Plants under Domestication.* New York: O. Judd and Co., 1868.

Delage, Yves, and Goldsmith, Marie. *The Theories of Evolution.* Trans. André Tridon. New York: B. W. Huebsch, 1913.

Diehl, Karl. "Johannes Conrad." *Jahrbücher für Nationalökonomie und Statistik* 104 (1915):737–762.

Diepgen, Paul. "Krankheitswesen und Krankheitsursachen in der spekulativen Pathologie des 19. Jahrhunderts." *Sudhoffs Archiv* 18 (1926):302–327.

Dietrich, A. *Die Bedeutung der Vererbung für die Pathologie.* Tübingen: Franz Pietzcker, 1902.

Dingfelder, Johannes. "Beitrag zur Vererbung erworbener Eigenschaften." *Biologisches Zentralblatt* 7 (1887–1888):427–432, 8 (1888–1889):210–217.

Dohrn, Schelle A. "Beiträge zur Lehre von Degenerationszeichen." *Deutsche zahnärztliche Wochenschrift* 8 (1906):97–98, 110–114, 125–127, 141–144.

Donath, J. "Die physische Degeneration der Bevölkerung in den modernen Culturstaaten mit besonderer Rücksicht auf Oesterreich-Ungarn." *Wiener medizinische Blätter* 17 (1894):537–538.

Earle, Pliny. *Institutions for the Insane in Prussia, Austria and Germany.* Utica, New York: New York State Lunatic Asylum, 1853.

Eibe, Th. "Referate über Psychiatrie." *Neurologisches Centralblatt* 7 (1888):448.

Enken, Rudolf, and Gruber, Max von. *Ethische und hygienische Aufgaben der Gegenwart.* Berlin: Mässigkeit, 1916.

Erb, Wilhelm. *Über die wachsende Nervosität unserer Zeit.* Heidelberg, Universitäts-Buchdruckerei von J. Hörning, 1893.

Die Erhaltung und Vermehrung der deutschen Volkskraft. Verhandlungen der 8. Konferenz der Zentralstelle für Volkswohlfahrt in Berlin vom 26. bis 28. Oktober 1915. Berlin: Heymann, 1916.

Eulenberg, F. "Degeneration der gebildeten Klassen." *Zeitschrift für die gesamten Staatswissenschaften* 61 (1905):353–367.

Eisler, Rudolf. *Wilhelm Wundts Philosophie und Psychologie.* Leipzig, Johann Ambrosius Barth, 1902.

Fahlbeck, Pontus. "Der Neo-Malthusianismus in seinen Beziehungen zur Rassenbiologie und Rassenhygiene." *ARGB* 8 (1912):30–48.

Fehlinger, Hans. *Rassenhygiene: Beiträge zur Entartungsfrage.* Langensalza: Wend und Klauwell, 1919.

Feilschenfeld, W. "Die Bestrebung der Eugenik in den Vereinigten Staaten von Nordamerika und ihre Übertragung auf deutsche Verhältnisse." *Medizinische Reform* 21 (1913):477–482.

Feld, Wilhelm. "Zur Statistik des Geburtenrückganges." *Conrads Jahrbücher für Nationalökonomie und Statistik* (1914):811–827.

Finke, Dr. "Biologische Aufgaben in der Kriminalpolitik." *Eugenik* 1 (1930):55–58.

Fircks, Arthur von. *Bevölkerungslehre und Bevölkerungspolitik.* Leipzig: C. L. Hirschfeld, 1898.

Fischer, Alfons. *Geschichte des deutschen Gesundheitswesens.* 2 vols. Berlin: F. A. Herbig, 1933.

Fischer, Eugen. "Aus der Geschichte der deutschen Gesellschaft für Rassenhygiene." *ARGB* 24 (1930):1–5.

———. "Sozialanthropologie." In *Handwörterbuch der naturwissenschaften,* 9:172–188. Jena: Gustav Fischer, 1912/13.

Forel, August. *Die sexuelle Frage.* 9th ed. Munich: Ernst Reinhardt, 1909.

Fuld, E. "Das rückfällige Verbrechertum." *Deutsche Zeit- und Streitfragen* 14 (1885):453–484.

Galton, Francis. "Experiments in Pangenesis by Breeding from Rabbits of a Pure Variety." *Proceedings of the Royal Society* (1871):393–410.

———. "Hereditary Improvement." *Fraser's Magazine* (Jan. 1873), 116–130.

———. *Genie und Verebung.* Trans. O. Neurath and A. Schapire-Neurath. Leipzig: W. Klinkhardt, 1910.

———. "The Possible Improvement of the Human Breed under the Existing Conditions of Law and Sentiment." *Nature* (1901):659–665.

———. *Essays in Eugenics.* London: The Eugenics Education Society, 1909.

Gaupp, Ernst. *August Weismann: Sein Leben und sein Werk.* Jena: Gustav Fischer, 1917.

Gaupp, Robert. "Über den heutigen Stand der Lehre von 'geborenen Verbrecher.'" *Monatsschrift für Kriminalpsychologie und Strafrechtsreform* (1904):25–42.

"Geleitwort." *Eugenik* 1 (1930), unpaginated.

Germany. Kaiserliches Statistisches Amt. *Statistisches Handbuch für das Deutsche Reich.* 2 vols. Berlin: Heymann, 1907.

———. Kaiserliche Gesundheits- und Statistische Ämter. *Das Deutsche Reich in gesundheitlicher und demographischer Beziehung. Festschrift den*

Theilnehmern am XIV. Internationalen Kongresse für Hygiene und Demographie, Berlin 1907. Berlin: Puttkammer und Mühlbrecht, 1907.

——. Reichsgesundheitsamt. *Das Reichsgesundheitsamt 1876–1926.* Berlin: Julius Springer, 1926.

——. Reichskommission, Internationale Hygiene-Ausstellung, Dresden, 1930–1931. *Die Entwicklung des deutschen Gesundheitswesens.* Berlin: Arbeitsgemeinschaft sozialhygienischer Reichsfachverbände, 1931.

Gerhardt, J. P. *Zur Geschichte und Literatur des Idiotenwesens in Deutschland.* Hamburg: privately published, 1904.

Gerstenhauer, M. R. "Rassenverfall durch Zivilisation und seine Bekämpfung." *Deutsche Tageszeitung,* 20 May 1912.

Gottstein, Adolf. "Die Entwicklung der Hygiene im letzten Vierteljahrhundert." *Zeitschrift für Sozialwissenschaft* 12 (1909):65–82.

Grassmann, K. "Kritische Ueberblick über die gegenwärtige Lehre von der Erblichkeit der Psychosen." *Allgemeine Zeitschrift für Psychiatrie* 52 (1896):960–1022.

Grotjahn, Alfred. *Geburtenrückgang und Geburtenregelung.* Berlin: Louis Marcus, 1914.

——. "Soziale Hygiene und Entartungsproblem." In *Handbuch der Hygiene.* Ed. Th. Weyl. 4th suppl. vol.: 727–789. Jena: Gustav Fischer, 1904.

Grotjahn, Alfred, and Kaup, J., eds. *Handwörterbuch der sozialen Hygiene.* Leipzig, F. C. W. Vogel, 1912.

Gruber, Max von. "Deutsche Gesundheitspflege." *Deutsche Revue* 43 (1918):64–78.

——. "Führt die Hygiene zur Entartung der Rasse?" *Münchener medizinische Wochenschrift* 50 (1903):1713–1718, 1781–1785.

——. *Ursachen und Bekämpfung des Geburtenrückganges im Deutschen Reich.* Munich: J. F. Lehmann, 1914.

——. "Vererbung, Auslese und Hygiene." *Deutsche Medizinische Wochenschrift* 46 (1909):1993–1996, 2049–2053.

——. "Wilhelm Schallmayer." *ARGB* 14 (1922):52–56.

Gruber, Max von, and Rüdin, Ernst. *Fortpflanzung, Vererbung, Rassenhygiene.* Munich: J. F. Lehmann, 1911.

Gütt, Arthur. "Ausmerze und Lebensauslese in ihre Bedeutung für Erbgesundheit und Rassenpflege." In *Erblehre und Rassenhygiene im völkischen Staat,* ed. Ernst Rüdin, 104–119. Munich: Lehmann, 1932.

Haeckel, Ernst. *Freedom in Science and Teaching.* New York: D. Appleton, 1879.

————. *The History of Creation: Or the Development of the Earth and Its Inhabitants by the Action of Natural Causes.* Trans. and rev. by E. Ray Lankester. London: Henry S. King and Co., 1876.

Hall, G. Stanley. *Founders of Modern Psychology.* New York: D. Appleton and Co., 1912.

Haycraft, John B. *Darwinism and Race Progress.* London: Swan Sonnenschein and Co., 1895.

Hegar, A. "Brüste und Stillen." *Deutsche medizinische Wochenschrift* 22 (1896):539–541.

Helmut, Otto. *Volk in Gefahr: Der Geburtenrückgang und seine Folgen für Deutschlands Zukunft.* Munich: J. F. Lehmann, 1934.

Hentig, Hans von. *Strafrecht und Auslese.* Berlin: J. Springer, 1914.

Herkner, Heinrich. "Die Entartungsfrage in England." *Schmollers Jahrbuch für Gesetzgebung und Verwaltung* 31 (1907):357–378.

Hertwig, Oscar. *Zur Abwehr des ethischen, des sozialen, des politischen Darwinismus.* 2d ed. Jena: Gustav Fischer, 1922.

Herz, Friedrich. *Rasse und Kultur.* 2d ed. of *Moderne Rassentheorien.* Leipzig: Alfred Kröner, 1915.

Hieronymus, D. "Vererbung und erbliche Belastung in ihrer Bedeutung für Jugend- und Volkserziehung." *Kinderfehler* 9 (1904):241–253.

Hitze, Franz. *Geburtenrückgang und Sozialreform.* Munich: M. Gladbacher Volksverein, 1917.

Hoffmann, G. von. "Eugenics in Germany: Society of Race Hygiene Adopts Resolution Calling for Extensive Program of Positive Measures to Check Decline in Birth-Rate." *Journal of Heredity* 5 (1914):435–436.

————. *Die Rassenhygiene in den Vereinigten Staaten von Nordamerika.* Munich: J. F. Lehmann, 1913.

Holmes, Samuel. *A Bibliography of Eugenics.* University of California Publications in Zoology, vol. 24. Berkeley: University of California Press, 1924.

Hueppe, E. Rev. of *Vererbung und Auslese,* by W. Schallmayer. *Zeitschrift für Sozialwissenschaft* 8 (1905):127–131.

Jörger, J. "Die Familie Zero." *ARGB* 2 (1905):494–559.

Johannsen, Wilhelm L. *Elementen der exakten Erblichkeitslehre.* Jena: Gustav Fischer, 1909.

Kaup, J. "Was kosten die minderwertigen Elemente dem Staat und der Gesellschaft?" *ARGB* 10 (1913):723–748.

Kautsky, Karl. Rev. of *Über die drohende körperliche Entartung der Kulturmenschheit,* by W. Schallmayer. *Die neue Zeit* 10 (1892):644–651.

Kellog, Vernon L. *Darwinism Today.* New York: Henry Holt, 1907.

Kende, Moriz. *Die Entartung des Menschengeschlechts, ihre Ursachen und die Mittel zu ihrer Bekämpfung.* Halle: Carl Marhold, 1901.

Knieke, H. "Die Verstaatlichung des Aerztewesens." *Politisch-anthropologische Revue* 2 (1903–1904):402–409.

Kraepelin, Emil. "Bernhard von Gudden." *Münchener medizinische Wochenschrift* 33 (1886):577–607.

Krafft-Ebing, Richard Freiherr von. *Lehrbuch der Psychiatrie.* 4th ed. Stuttgart: Ferdinand Enke, 1890.

———. "Nervosität und neurasthenische Zustände." In *Specielle Pathologie und Therapie,* ed. Hermann Nothnagel, 2, pt. 2:1–210. Vienna: Alfred Holder, 1899.

———. *Über gesunde und kranke Nerven.* Tübingen: Laupp'sche Buchhandlung, 1885.

Kresse, Oskar. *Der Geburtenrückgang in Deutschland, seine Ursachen und die Mittel zu seiner Beseitigung.* Berlin: John Schwerin, 1912.

Kruse, Walter. "Entartung." *Zeitschrift für Sozialwissenschaft* 6 (1903):359–376.

———. "Physische Degeneration und Wehrfähigkeit bei europäischen Völkern." *Zentralblatt für allgemeine Gesundheitspflege* 17 (1898):457–473.

Kuhlenbeck, Ludwig. "Kritik der Jenaser Preisschriften." *Politisch-anthropologischen Revue* 3 (1904–1905):427–435.

Kurella, Hans. *Naturgeschichte des Verbrechers: Grundzüge der criminellen Anthropologie und Criminalpsychologie.* Stuttgart: Ferdinand Enke, 1893.

Lapouge, Georges Vacher de. "Kritik des Jenenser Preisauschreibens." *Politisch-anthropologischer Revue* 3 (1904–1905):297–304.

———. "Ludwig Woltmann, ein Bahnbrecher der Sozialanthropologie." *Politisch-anthropologische Revue* 6 (1907–1908):37–41.

———. "Ueber die natürliche Minderwertigkeit der modernen Bevölkerungsklassen." *Politisch-anthropologische Revue* 8 (1909–1910):393–409, 454–464.

Lenz, Fritz. "Alfred Ploetz zum 70. Geburtstag." *ARGB* 24 (1930):viii–xv.

———. "Bevölkerungspolitik und 'Mutterschutz.'" *ARGB* 12 (1916–1918):345–348.

———. "Deutsche Gesellschaft für Bevölkerungspolitik." *ARGB* 11 (1914–1915):555–557.

———. Rev. of "Einführung in die Rassehygiene," by W. Schallmayer. *Münchener medizinische Wochenschrift* 64 (1917):554.

———. "Notizen." *ARGB* 12 (1916–1918):116–124.

———. "Rassenhygienische Bevölkerungspolitik." *Deutsche Politik* 1 (1916):1658–1668.

———. "Überblick über die Rassenhygiene." *Jahreskurse für ärztliche Fortbildung* 8 (1917):16–50.

———. "Vorschläge zur Bevölkerungspolitik mit besonderer Berücksichtigung der Wirtschaftslage nach dem Kriege." *ARGB* 12 (1916–1918):440–468.

———. "Wilhelm Schallmayer." *Münchener medizinische Wochenschrift* 66 (1919):1294–1296.

———. "Zum Begriff der Rassenhygiene und seine Benennung." *ARGB* 11 (1914–1915):445–448.

———. "Zur Erneuerung der Ethik." *Deutschlands Erneuerung* (1917):35–56.

Löwenfeld, Leopold. *Pathologie und Therapie der Neurasthenie und Hysterie.* Wiesbaden: J. F. Bergmann, 1894.

———. "Über medizinische Schutzmaßnahmen gegen Verbrechen." *Sexualprobleme* (1910):300–327.

Magnus-Levy, Adolf. "The Heroic Age of German Medicine." *Bulletin of the History of Medicine* 16 (1944):331–342.

Marcuse, Julian. *Die Beschränkung der Geburtenzahl: Ein Kulturproblem.* Munich: E. Reinhardt, 1913.

Marcuse, Max. "Gesetzliche Eheverbote für Kranke und Minderwertige." *Soziale Medizin und Hygiene* 2 (1907):96–108, 163–175.

———. "Die Verhütung der Geisteskrankheiten durch Eheverbote." *Allgemeine Zeitung* (Munich), 13 June 1908.

Martius, Friedrich. "Die Bedeutung der Vererbung für Krankheitsentstehung und Rassenerhaltung." *ARGB* 7 (1910):470–489.

———. *Konstitution und Vererbung in ihren Beziehungen zur Pathologie.* Berlin: J. Springer, 1914.

———. "Künstliche Fehlgeburt und künstliche Unfruchtbarkeit vom Standpunkt der inneren Medizin." In *Künstliche Fehlgeburt und künstliche Unfruchtbarkeit: Ihre Indikationen, Technik und Rechtlage,* ed. Siegfied Placzek, 49–120. Leipzig: G. Thieme, 1918.

———. *Neurasthenische Entartung einst und jetzt.* Leipzig and Vienna: Franz Deuticke, 1909.

———. "Die Vererbbarkeit des constitutionellen Faktors der Tuberculose." *Berliner klinische Wochenschrift* 38 (1901):1125–1130.

———. "Das Vererbungsproblem in der Pathologie." *Berliner klinische Wochenschrift* 38 (1901):781–783, 814–818.

Meyer, Ludwig. "Die Zunahme der Geisteskrankheiten." *Deutsche Rundschau* (1885):78–94.

Möbius, Paul Julius. *Die Nervosität*. Leipzig: J. J. Weber, 1882.

————. *Ueber Entartung*. Wiesbaden: J. F. Bergmann, 1900.

Mönkemöller, Eduard Otto. "Kriminalität." In *Handwörterbuch der sozialen Hygiene*, ed. A. Grotjahn and J. Kaup. Leipzig: F. C. W. Vogel, 1912.

Morel, Bénédict A. *Traité des dégénérescences physiques, intellectuelles et morales de l'espèce humaine*. Paris: J. B. Bailliere, 1857.

Muckermann, Hermann. "Illustrationen zu der Frage: Wohlfahrtspflege und Eugenik." *Eugenik* 2 (1931):41–42.

————. *Volkstum, Staat und Nation, eugenisch gesehen*. Essen: Fredebeul und Koenen, 1933.

————, and Verschuer, O. Freiherr von. *Eugenische Eheberatung*. Berlin: Dümmler, 1931.

Müller, Franz Carl, ed. *Handbuch der Neurasthenie*. Leipzig: F. C. W. Vogel, 1893.

Näcke, Paul. "Die ersten Kastrationen aus sozialen Gründen auf europäischen Boden." *Neurologisches Zentralblatt* (1909):226–234.

————. "Kastration bei gewissen Klassen von Degenerierten als ein wirksamer sozialer Schutz." *Archiv für Kriminalanthropologie* 1 (1899):58–84.

————. "Über den Wert der sogenannten Degenerationszeichen." *Monatsschrift für Kriminalpsychologie und Strafrechtsreform* 1 (1904):99–111.

————. *Verbrechen und Wahnsinn beim Weibe*. Vienna and Leipzig: Wilhelm Braumüller, 1894.

Nef, Willy. *Die Philosophie Wilhelm Wundts*. Leipzig: Felix Meiner, 1923.

Nordenskiöld, Erik. *The History of Biology*. Trans. Leonard Bucknell Eyre. New York: Tudor, 1928.

Oettingen, Alexander K. von. *Die Moralstatistik in ihrer Bedeutung für eine Sozialethik*. 3d ed. Erlangen: A. Deichert, 1882.

Oettinger, W. "Selektion und Hygiene." *Deutsche Vierteljahrsschrift für öffentliche Gesundheitspflege* (1912):608–626.

Olberg, Oda. "Bemerkungen über Rassenhygiene und Sozialismus." *Die neue Zeit* 25 (1906):725–733.

————. "Rassenhygiene und Sozialismus." *Die neue Zeit* 26 (1907):882–887.

Oldenberg, K. "Der Geburtenrückgang und seine treibenden Kräfte." *Deutschlands Erneuerung* (1918):264–279.

————. "Über den Rückgang der Geburten- und Sterbeziffer." *Archiv für Sozialwissenschaft und Sozialpolitik* (1911):319–377.

Orth, J. "Ueber die Entstehung und Vererbung individueller Eigenschaften." In *Festschrift Albert von Kölliker zur Feier seines siebzigsten Geburtstages*, 157–183. Leipzig: Wilhelm Engelmann, 1887.

Pearson, Karl. *The Scope and Importance to the State of the Science of National Eugenics.* 3d ed. London: Cambridge University Press, 1911.

Peltzer, Otto. "Das Verhältnis der Sozialpolitik zur Rassenhygiene: Eine kritische Studie über die Auswirkung biologischer Erkenntnisse auf die Lösungsversuche sozialer Probleme." Diss., Munich, 1925/26.

Plate, Ludwig. *Die Bedeutung und Tragweite des Darwinischen Selektionsprinzipes.* Leipzig: W. Engelmann, 1900.

Ploetz, Alfred. "Ableitung einer Gesellschaftshygiene und ihrer Beziehung zur Ethik." *ARGB* 3 (1906):253–260.

————. "Ableitung einer Rassenhygiene und ihrer Beziehung zur Ethik." *Vierteljahresschrift für wissenschaftliche Philosophie* 19 (1895):368–377.

————. "Der Alkohol im Lebensprozess der Rasse." *Internationale Monatsschrift zur Erforschung des Alkoholismus und Bekämpfung der Trunksitten* (1903):239–289.

————. "Die Begriffe Rasse und Gesellschaft und die davon abgeleiteten Disciplinen." *ARGB* 1 (1904):2–26.

————. "Die Begriffe Rasse und Gesellschaft und einige damit zusammenhängende Probleme." *Schriften der deutschen Gesellschaft für Soziologie* 1 (1911):111–136.

————. "Kritik über Max von Gruber: 'Führt die Hygiene zur Entartung der Rasse.'" *ARGB* 1 (1904):157.

————. "Neo-Malthusianismus und Rassenhygiene." *ARGB* 10 (1913):166–172.

————. "Rassentüchtigkeit und Sozialismus." *Neue Deutsche Rundschau* 5 (1894):989–997.

————. "Sozialpolitik und Rassenhygiene in ihrem prinzipiellen Verhältnis." *Archiv für soziale Gesetzgebung und Statistik* 17 (1902):393–420.

————. "Trostworte an einem naturwissenschaftlichen Hamlet." Reprint of an article in the *New Yorker Volkszeitung*, 6 Nov. 1892. *ARGB* 29 (1935):88–89.

————. *Die Tüchtigkeit unsrer Rasse und der Schutz der Schwachen. Ein Versuch über Rassenhygiene und ihr Verhältnis zu den humanen Idealen, besonders zum Socialismus.* Berlin: Gustav Fischer, 1895.

———. "Ziele und Aufgabe der Rassenhygiene." *Vierteljahrsschrift für öffentliche Gesundheitspflege* 43 (1911):164–191.

———. "Zur Abgrenzung und Einleitung des Begriffs Rassenhygiene." *ARGB* 3 (1906):864–866.

———. Nordenholz, Anastasius, and Plate, Ludwig. "Vorwort." *ARGB* 1 (1904):iii–vi.

Potthoff, Heinz. "Schutz der Schwachen." *ARGB* 8 (1911):86–91.

Prinzing, Friedrich. "Die angebliche Wirkung hoher Kindersterblichkeit im Sinne Darwinscher Auslese." *Zentralblatt für allgemeine Gesundheitspflege* (1903):111–129.

Rahm, Hermann. "Deszendenztheorie und Sozialrecht." *Annalen des deutschen Reiches* (1906):703–717.

Reibmayr, Albert. "Die biologischen Gefahren der heutigen Frauenemanzipation." *Politisch-anthropologische Revue* 5 (1906–1907):445–468.

———. *Die Entwicklungsgeschichte des Talentes und Genies.* Munich: J. F. Lehmann, 1908.

Reich, Eduard. *Über die Entartung des Menschen, ihre Ursachen und Verhütung.* Erlangen: Ferdinand Enke, 1868.

Ribbert, Hugo. *Rassenhygiene: Eine gemeinverständliche Darstellung.* Bonn: Friedrich Cohen, 1910.

Ribot, Théodule Armand. *Heredity: A Psychological Study of Its Phenomena, Laws, Causes, and Consequences.* New York: D. Appleton and Co., 1875.

Rubin, Marcus and Westergaard, Harald. *Statistik der Ehen auf Grund der sozialen Gliederung der Bevölkerung.* Jena: Gustav Fischer, 1890.

Rüdin, Ernst. "Über den Zusammenhang zwischen Geisteskrankheit und Kultur." *ARGB* 7 (1910):722–748.

———. "20 Jahre menschliche Erbforschung an der Deutschen Forschungsanstalt für Psychiatrie in München, Kaiser Wilhelm-Institut." *ARGB* 32 (1938): 193–203.

Rutgers, Johannes. *Rassenverbesserung, Malthusianismus und Neumalthusianismus.* Trans. Martina G. Kramers. Dresden and Leipzig: Heinrich Minden, 1908.

Samuelsohn, J. "Zur Genese der angeborenen Mißbildungen, speciell des Microphthalmus congenitus." *Zentralblatt für medizinische Wissenschaft* 18 (1880):305–308, 322–324.

Samson-Himmelstjerna, Hermann von. *Die gelbe Gefahr als Moralproblem.* Berlin: Deutscher Kolonial Verlag, 1902.

Schallmayer, Otto. "Wilhelm Schallmayer." *Akademischer Gesangverein* (1919 or 1920):1–4.

Scheidt, Walter. "Beiträge zur Geschichte der Anthropologie: Der Begriff Rasse in der Anthropologie und die Einteilung der Menschenrassen von Linné bis Deniker." *ARGB* 15 (1923):280–306, 383–397; 16 (1924):178–202, 382–403.

Schemann, Ludwig. *Gobineaus Rassenwerk: Aktenstücke und Betrachtungen zur Geschichte und Kritik des Essai sur l'inégalité des races humaines.* Stuttgart: Fromann, 1910.

———. "Wilhelm Schallmayer." *Politisch-anthropologische Monatsschrift* 18 (1919–1920):469–471.

Schmoller, Gustav. *Die soziale Frage und der preussische Staat.* Munich and Leipzig: Duncker und Humblot, 1918.

Schneider, K. V. "Über den heutigen Stand der Deszendenztheorie." *Wiener klinische Rundschau* 18 (1904):78–81, 99–101, 115–117.

Schopol, Dr., ed. *Die Eugenik im Dienste der Volkswohlfahrt. Bericht über die Verhandlungen eines zusammengesetzten Ausschusses des Preussischen Landesgesundheitsrats vom 2. Juli 1932.* Veröffentlichungen aus dem Gebiete der Medizinalverwaltung, XXXVIII. Band—5. Heft. Berlin: Richard Schoetz, 1932.

Seeberg, Reinhold. *Der Geburtenrückgang in Deutschland, eine sozialethische Studie.* Leipzig: A. Deichert, 1913.

Seeck, Otto. *Geschichte des Untergangs der antiken Welt.* 6 vols. 1920–1922. Reprint. Darmstadt: Wissenschaftliche Buchgesellschaft, 1966.

Siemens, Hermann W. *Die biologischen Grundlagen der Rassenhygiene und der Bevölkerungspolitik.* Munich: J. F. Lehmann, 1917.

———. "Biologische Terminologie und rassenhygienische Propaganda." *ARGB* 12 (1916–1918):257–267.

———. "Die Familie Siemens." *ARGB* 11 (1914–1915):486–489.

———. "Kritik der Rassenhygiene." *Politisch-anthropologische Monatsschrift* 15 (1916–1917):30–48, 98–104, 158–164.

———. "Kritik der rassenhygienischen und bevölkerungspolitischen Bestrebungen." *Politisch-anthropologische Monatsschrift* 15 (1916–1917): 547–551.

———. "Die Proletarisierung unseres Nachwuchses, eine Gefahr unrassenhygienischer Bevölkerungspolitik." *ARGB* 12 (1916–1918):43–55.

———. "Wilhelm Schallmayers Vererbung und Auslese." *ARGB* 14 (1922):75–77.

Sigerist, Henry E. "Das Bild des Menschen in der modernen Medizin." *Neue Blätter für den Sozialismus* 1 (1930):97–106.

Siol, E. "Über direkte Vererbung von Geisteskrankheiten." *Archiv für Psychiatrie und Nervenkrankheiten* 16 (1885):113–150, 353–409, 599–638.

Sombart, Werner. "Ideale der Sozialpolitik." *Archiv für soziale Gesetzgebung und Statistik* 10 (1897):1–48.

Spencer, Herbert. *Essays Scientific, Political and Speculative.* Library ed., I. New York: D. Appleton and Co., 1891.

Steinmetz, Sebald R. "Die erbliche Rassen- und Volkscharakter." *Vierteljahrsschrift für wissenschaftliche Philosophie und Soziologie* (1902): 77–126.

———. Rev. of *Vererbung und Auslese,* by W. Schallmayer. *Vierteljahrsschrift für wissenschaftliche Philosophie und Soziologie* (1906): 115–116.

———. Rev. of *Vererbung und Auslese,* by W. Schallmayer. *Zeitschrift für Sozialwissenschaft,* N. F., 1 (1910):1817–1818.

———. "Feminismus und Rasse." *Zeitschrift für Sozialwissenschaft* 7 (1904):751–768.

———. "Der Nachwuchs der Begabten." *Zeitschrift für Sozialwissenschaft* 7 (1904):1–25.

———. *Die Philosophie des Krieges.* Leipzig: Johann Ambrosius Barth, 1907.

Stern, William. *Die psychologischen Methoden der Intelligenzprüfung und deren Anwendung an Schulkindern.* Leipzig: Johann Ambrosius Barth, 1912.

Strangeland, Charles E. *Pre-Malthusian Doctrines of Population: A Study in the History of Economic Theory.* 1904. Reprint. New York: Augustus M. Kelley, 1966.

Tille, Alexander. *Von Darwin bis Nietzsche: Ein Buch Entwicklungsethik.* Leipzig: C. G. Naumann, 1895.

Thomsen, J. "Beobachtung über Trunksucht und ihre Erblichkeit." *Archiv für Psychiatrie* 17 (1886):527–546.

Tönnies, Ferdinand. "Ammons Gesellschaftstheorie." *Zeitschrift für Sozialwissenschaft* 7 (1904):88–111.

———. "Eugenik." *Schmollers Jahrbuch für Gesetzgebung und Verwaltung* 29 (1903):273–290.

———. "Zur naturwissenschaftlichen Gesellschaftslehre." *Schmollers Jahrbuch für Gesetzgebung und Verwaltung* 31 (1905):27–102, 1283–1321.

———. "Zur naturwissenschaftlichen Gesellschaftslehre: Eine Replik." *Schmollers Jahrbuch für Gesetzgebung und Verwaltung* 33 (1907):49–114.

"Ueber die drohende körperliche Entartung der Culturmenschheit und die Verstaatlichung des ärztlichen Standes." *Münchener medizinische Wochenschrift* 27 (1892):478–480.

"Über die Vererbung von Geisteskrankheiten nach Beobachtung in preussischen Irrenanstalten." *Jahrbuch für Psychiatrie und Neurologie* 1 (1879):65–66.

Verhandlungen des Ersten Deutschen Soziologentages. Tübingen: J. C. B. Mohr, 1911.

Verschuer, Otto Freiherr von. *Leitfaden der Rassenhygiene.* Leipzig: Georg Thieme, 1941.

Vierkandt, A. "Ein Einbruch der Naturwissenschaften in die Geisteswissenschaften?" *Zeitschrift für philosophische Kritik* 127 (1906):168–177.

————. Rev. of *Vererbung und Auslese,* by W. Schallmayer. *Archiv für die gesamte Psychologie* 7 (1906):183–185.

Virchow, Rudolf. "Descendenz und Pathologie." *Virchows Archiv für pathologische Anatomie und Physiologie und für klinische Medizin* 103 (1886):1–14.

————. *The Freedom of Science in the Modern State.* 2d ed. London: John Murray, 1878.

Voss, G. "Zur Frage der Entartung und des Entartungirreseins." *Deutsche medizinische Wochenschrift* 36 (1910):25–28.

Wagner, Adolph. *Rede über die sociale Frage.* Berlin: Wiegandt und Grieben, 1872.

Wahl, M. "Über den gegenwärtigen Stand der Erblichkeitsfrage in der Lehre von der Tuberculose." *Deutsche medizinische Wochenschrift* (1885), no. 1:3–5; no. 3:36–38; no. 4:34–56, no. 5:69–71, no. 6:88–90.

Wallace, Alfred R. *Contributions to the Theory of Natural Selection: A Series of Essays.* London, Macmillan, 1875.

————. *Darwinism: An Exposition of the Theory of Natural Selection with Some of its Applications.* London: Macmillan, 1889.

————. "Are Individually Acquired Characters Inherited." In *Studies Scientific and Social.* London: Macmillan, 1875.

————. "Menschheitsfortschritt." *Die Zukunft* 8 (1894):145–158.

————. "Menschliche Auslese." *Die Zukunft* 8 (1894):10–24.

————. "The Method of Organic Evolution." In *Smithsonian Institution Annual Report.* Washington: U. S. Government Printing Office, 1894.

Weigert, C. "Neuere Vererbungstheorien." *Schmidts Jahrbücher der gesammten Medizin* (1887):89–104, 193–206.

Weismann, August. "The All-Sufficiency of Natural Selection: A Reply to Herbert Spencer." *Contemporary Review* 64 (1893):309–338, 596–610.

―――. *Essays Upon Heredity and Kindred Problems.* Eds. Edward Poulton, Selmar Schönland, and Arthur Shipley. Oxford: Clarendon, 1889.

―――. *Neue Gedanken zur Vererbungsfrage: Eine Antwort an Herbert Spencer.* Jena: Gustav Fischer, 1895.

―――. *Über Germinal-Selektion: Eine Quelle bestimmt gerichteter Variation.* Jena: Gustav Fischer, 1896.

―――. "Über den Rückschritt in der Natur." *Deutsche Rundschau* 48 (1886):437–459.

―――. *Über die Berechtigung der Darwin'schen Theorie.* Leipzig: Engelmann, 1868.

―――. *Vorträge über Deszendenztheorie.* 2 vols. 2d ed. Jena: Gustav Fischer, 1904.

Wer Ist's. 8th ed. Leipzig: Ludwig Degener, 1914.

Wolf, Julius. *Der Geburtenrückgang.* Jena: Gustav Fischer, 1912.

Woltmann, Ludwig. "Nachschrift zu Lapouges Kritik des Jeneser Preisausschreibens." *Politisch-anthropologische Revue* 3 (1904–1905): 305–317.

―――. *Politische Anthropologie: Eine Untersuchung über den Einfluß der Deszcendenztheorie auf der Lehre von der politischen Entwicklung der Völker.* Leipzig and Eisenach: Anst, 1903.

―――. "Die Preisrichter von Jena." *Politisch-anthropologische Revue* 4 (1905–1906):48–51.

Ziegler, Heinrich Ernst. "Einleitung zu dem Sammelwerke *Natur und Staat.*" In *Natur und Staat: Beiträge zur naturwissenschaftlichen Gesellschaftslehre.* Jena: Gustav Fischer, 1903.

―――. Rev. of *Vererbung und Auslese,* by W. Schallmayer. *Deutsche Literaturzeitung* (1904):681–685.

―――. *Die Naturwissenschaft und die socialdemokratische Theorie, ihr Verhältnis dargelegt auf Grund der Werke von Darwin und Bebel.* Stuttgart: Enke, 1893.

―――. *Über den derzeitigen Stand der Descendenztheorie in der Zoologie.* Jena: Gustav Fischer, 1902.

―――. *Die Vererbungslehre in der Biologie.* Jena: Gustav Fischer, 1905.

―――. *Die Vererbungslehre in der Biologie und in der Soziologie.* Jena: Gustav Fischer, 1918.

―――. "Das Verhältnis der Sozialdemokratie zum Darwinismus." *Zeitschrift für Sozialwissenschaft* 2 (1899):424–432.

―――. "Wilhelm Schallmayer." *Deutsche medizinische Wochenschrift* (1920):1–3.

————. "Zu den Kritiken über das Jeneser Preisausschreiben." *Politisch-anthropologische Revue* 3 (1904–1905):436–448.

PUBLICATIONS AFTER 1945

Ackerknecht, Erwin H. *A Short History of Psychiatry.* Trans. Sula Wolff. 2d ed. New York and London: Hafner, 1968.

Allen, Garland. "The Eugenics Record Office at Cold Spring Harbor, 1910–1940: An Essay in Institutional History." *Osiris,* 2d series, 2 (1986):225–264.

————. "Genetics, Eugenics and Society: Internalists and Externalists in Contemporary History of Science." *Social Studies of Science* 6 (1976):105–122.

————. "A History of Eugenics in the Class Struggle." *Science for the People* 6 (1974):32–37, 39.

Altner, Günter. *Weltanschauliche Hintergründe der Rassenlehrer des Dritten Reiches.* Zurich: EVZ, 1968.

Artelt, Walter, et. al., eds. *Städte-, Wohnungs- und Kleidungshygiene des 19. Jahrhunderts in Deutschland.* Stuttgart: Ferdinand Enke, 1969.

Baader, Gerhard. "Das 'Gesetz zur Verhütung erbkranken Nachwuchses'—Versuch einer kritischen Deutung." In *Zusammenhang. Festschrift für Marielene Putscher,* ed. Otto Baur and Otto Glandien, 865–875. Cologne: Wienand, 1984.

————, and Schultz, Ulrich, eds. *Medizin und Nationalsozialismus: Tabuisierte Vergangenheit—Ungebrochene Tradition?* Dokumentation des Gesundheitstages Berlin 1980, I. Berlin-West: Verlagsgesellschaft Gesundheit mbH., 1980.

Bade, Klaus J. "German Emigration to the United States and Continental Immigration to Germany in the Late Nineteenth and Early Twentieth Centuries." *Central European History* 13 (1980):348–377.

Baitsch, Helmut. "Das eugenische Konzept einst und jetzt." In *Genetik und Gesellschaft,* ed. G. Wendt, 59–71. Stuttgart: Wissenschaftliche Verlagsgesellschaft mbH, 1970.

Bajema, Carl, ed. *Eugenics: Then and Now.* Strandsberg, Pa.: Dowden, Hutchinson and Ross, 1976.

Baker, John R. *Race.* London: Oxford University Press, 1974.

Barraclough, Geoffrey. *An Introduction to Contemporary History.* New York: Penguin, 1981.

Beckwith, John. "Social and Political Uses of Genetics in the United

States: Past and Present." *Annals of the New York Academy of Sciences* 256 (1976): 46–58.

Bender, Donald. "The Development of French Anthropology." *Journal of the Behavioral Sciences* 1 (1965):139–151.

Benz, Ernst. *Der Übermensch: Eine Diskussion.* Stuttgart: Rhein, 1961.

Berghahn, Volker R. *Germany and the Approach of War in 1914.* London: Macmillan, 1973.

Biddiss, Michael D. *Father of Racist Theory: The Social and Political Thought of Count Gobineau.* London and New York: Weybright and Talley, 1970.

Blacker, Charles P. *Eugenics. Galton and After.* London: Duckworth, 1952.

Blasius, Dirk. "Kriminalität als Gegenstand historischer Forschung." *Kriminalsoziologische Bibiliographie* 6 (1979):1–15.

Bock, Gisela. *Zwangssterilisation im Nationalsozialismus. Studien zur Rassenpolitik und Frauenpolitik.* Schriften des Zentralinstituts für sozialwissenschaftliche Forschung der Freien Universität Berlin, Bd. 48. Opladen: Westdeutscher Verlag, 1986.

———. "Racism and Sexism in Nazi Germany: Motherhood, Compulsory Sterilization and the State." In *When Biology Became Destiny: Women in Weimar and Nazi Germany,* ed. Renate Bridenthal, Atina Grossmann, and Marion Kaplan, 271–296. New York: Monthly Review Press, 1984.

Bolle, Fritz. "Darwinismus und Zeitgeist." *Zeitschrift für Religions- und Geistesgeschichte* 14 (1962):143–178.

Bowler, Peter J. *The Eclipse of Darwinism: Anti-Darwinian Evolution Theories in the Decades around 1900.* Baltimore: Johns Hopkins University Press, 1983.

———. *Evolution: The History of an Idea.* Berkeley, Los Angeles, London: University of California Press, 1984.

Breiling, Rupert. *Die nationalsozialistische Rassenlehre. Entstehung, Ausbreitung, Nutzen und Schaden einer politischen Ideologie.* Meisenheim am Glan: Anton Hain, 1971.

Burgener, Peter. *Die Einflüsse des zeitgenossischen Denkens in Morels Begriff der dégénérescence.* Zürcher medizingeschichtliche Abhandlungen, no. 16. Zurich: Juris, 1964.

Burkhardt, Claudia. *Euthanasie—"Vernichtung lebensunwerten Lebens" im Spiegel der Diskussion zwischen Juristen und Medizinern von 1900 bis 1940.* Med. diss., Mainz, 1981. Mainz: privately printed, 1981.

Chase, Allan. *The Legacy of Malthus.* New York: Alfred A. Knopf, 1977.

Chorover, Stephan L. *From Genesis to Genocide: The Meaning of Human*

Nature and the Power of Behavior Control. Cambridge, Mass.: MIT Press, 1979.

Churchill, Fredrick. "August Weismann and a Break From Tradition." *Journal of the History of Biology* 1 (1968):91–112.

————. "Rudolf Virchow and the Pathologist's Criteria for the Inheritance of Acquired Characteristics." *Journal of the History of Medicine* 31 (1976):117–148.

Clark, Linda L. *Social Darwinism in France.* University, Ala.: The University of Alabama Press, 1984.

Conrad-Martius, Hedwig. *Utopien der Menschenzüchtung: Der Sozialdarwinismus und seine Folgen.* Munich: Kösel, 1955.

Corning, Constance. "Francis Galton and Eugenics." *History Today* 23 (1973):724–732.

Cowan, Ruth Schwartz. "Nature and Nurture: The Interplay of Biology and Politics in the Work of Francis Galton." *Studies in the History of Biology* 1 (1977):135–208.

————. "Francis Galton's Contribution to Genetics." *Journal of the History of Biology* 5 (1972):389–412.

Cravens, Hamilton. *The Triumph of Evolution: American Scientists and the Heredity-Environment Controversy 1900–1914.* Philadelphia: University of Pennsylvania Press, 1978.

Dahrendorf, Ralf. *Society and Democracy in Germany.* New York: Anchor, 1969.

Davin, Anna. "Imperialism and Motherhood." *History Workshop,* no. 5 (1978):9–65.

Deppe, Hans-Ulrich, and Regus, Michael, eds. *Seminar: Medizin, Gesellschaft, Geschichte. Beiträge zur Entwicklungsgeschichte der Medizinsoziologie.* Frankfurt: Suhrkamp, 1975.

Diepgen, Paul. *Geschichte der Medizin,* II, pt. 2. Berlin: Walter de Gruyter, 1955.

Dietl, Hans-Martin, et. al. *Eugenik. Entstehung und gesellschaftliche Bedingtheit.* Medizin und Gesellschaft, Bd. 22. Jena: VEB Gustav Fischer, 1984.

Doeleke, Werner. *Alfred Ploetz (1860–1940): Sozialdarwinist und Gesellschaftsbiologe.* Med. diss., Frankfurt, 1975. Tübingen: privately printed, 1975.

Dörner, Klaus. "Nationalsozialismus und Lebensvernichtung." *Vierteljahrshefte für Zeitgeschichte* 15 (1967):121–152.

Ebert, Hans. "Hermann Muckermann: Profil eines Theologen, Widerstandskämpfers und Hochschullehrers der Technischen Universität Berlin." *Humanismus und Technik* 20 (1976):29–40.

Evans, Richard. *The Feminist Movement in Germany 1894–1933.* Sage Studies in 20th Century History, 6. London and Beverly Hills: Sage, 1976.

———. "Prostitution, State and Society in Imperial Germany." *Past and Present,* no. 70 (1976):106–129.

———, ed. *Society and Politics in Wilhelmine Germany.* New York: Barnes and Noble, 1978.

Farrall, Lyndsay. "The History of Eugenics: A Bibliographical Review." *Annals of Science* 36 (1975):111–123.

———. "The Origins and Growth of the English Eugenics Movement 1865–1925." Ph.D. diss., Indiana University, 1970.

Fichtmüller, W. "Dissertationen in den medizinischen Fakultäten der Universitäten Deutschlands von 1933–1945 zum Thema: 'Gesetz zur Verhütung erbkranken Nachwuchses vom 14. Juli 1933.' " Med. diss., Erlangen-Nürnberg, 1972.

Firth, Raymond. "Social Anthropology." In *The International Encyclopedia of the Social Sciences,* 1–2:320–324. New York: Macmillan and the Free Press, 1968.

Fischer, Wolfram, and Bajor, George, eds. *Die soziale Frage.* Stuttgart: K. F. Koehler, 1967.

Foucault, Michel. *The History of Sexuality. Volume 1: An Introduction.* New York: Pantheon, 1978.

Freeden, Michael. "Eugenics and Progressive Thought: A Study in Ideological Affinity." *Historical Journal* 22 (1979):645–671.

Fremdling, Rainer. "Railroads and German Economic Growth: A Leading Sector Analysis with a Comparison to the United States and Great Britain." *Journal of Economic History* 37 (1977):583–604.

Friedlander, Ruth. "Bénédict Augustin Morel and the Development of the Theory of *dégénérescence.*" Ph.D. diss., University of San Francisco, 1973.

Gasman, Daniel. *The Scientific Origins of National Socialism: Social Darwinism in Ernst Haeckel and the German Monist League.* New York: American Elsevier, 1971.

Geison, G. L. "Darwin and Heredity: The Evolution of his Hypothesis of Pangenesis." *Journal of the History of Medicine* 24 (1969):375–411.

Gerlada, Alfred. "Untersuchungen zur Geschichte des *Archivs für Rassen- und Gesellschaftsbiologie.*" Unpub. paper, Johannes Gutenberg-Universität, Mainz, 1973/74.

Ghiselin, Michael T. *The Triumph of the Darwinian Method.* Berkeley and Los Angeles: University of California Press, 1969.

Gladen, Albin. *Geschichte der Sozialpolitik in Deutschland.* Wiesbaden: Steiner, 1974.

Glass, Bentley. "A Hidden Chapter of German Eugenics Between the Two World Wars." *Proceedings of the American Philosophical Society* 125 (1981):357–367.

Glick, Thomas F., ed. *The Comparative Reception of Darwin.* Austin: University of Texas Press, 1974.

Göckenjan, Gerd. *Kurieren und Staat machen, Gesundheit und Medizin in der bürgerlichen Welt.* Frankfurt am Main: Suhrkamp, 1985.

Gordon, Linda. *Woman's Body, Woman's Right: A Social History of Birth Control in America.* New York: Penguin, 1977.

Gosling, Francis G. "American Nervousness: A Study in Medicine and Social Values in the Gilded Age, 1870–1900." Ph.D. diss., University of Oklahoma, 1976.

Graham, Loren R. "Science and Values: The Eugenics Movement in Germany and Russia in the 1920s." *American Historical Review* 82 (1977):1133–1164.

Greene, John C. "Darwin as a Social Evolutionist." *Journal of the History of Biology* 10 (1977):1–27.

Günther, Maria. *Über die Konsituierung der Rassenhygiene an den deutschen Universitäten vor 1933.* Med. diss., Mainz, 1982. Mainz: privately printed, 1982.

Güse, Hans-Georg, and Schmacke, Norbert. *Psychiatrie zwischen bürgerlicher Revolution und Faschismus.* 2 vols. Hamburg: Athenäum, 1976.

Hafner, Karl Heinz, and Winau, Rolf. "'Die Freigabe der Vernichtung lebensunwerten Lebens': Eine Untersuchung zu der Schrift von Karl Binding und Alfred Hoche." *Medizinhistorisches Journal* 9 (1974): 227–254.

Haller, John S. "Neurasthenia: Medical Profession and Urban 'Blahs.'" *New York State Journal of Medicine* 70 (1970):2489–2496.

———. *Outcasts From Evolution: Scientific Attitudes of Racial Inferiority 1859–1900.* Urbana: University of Illinois Press, 1971.

Haller, Mark. *Eugenics: Hereditarian Attitudes in American Thought.* New Brunswick, N. J.: Rutgers University Press, 1963.

Halliday, R. "Social Darwinism: A Definition." *Victorian Studies* 14 (1971):389–405.

Herbert, Sandra. "Darwin, Malthus and Selection." *Journal of the History of Biology* 4 (1971):209–217.

Hoffmann, Walther G. "The Take-Off in Germany." In *The Economics of*

Take-Off into Sustained Growth, ed. W. W. Rostow. London: Macmillan, 1963.

Hohorst, Gerd; Kocka, Jürgen; and Ritter, Gerhard A. *Sozialgeschichtliches Arbeitsbuch. Materialien zur Statistik des Kaiserreichs 1870–1914.* Munich: C. H. Beck, 1975.

Huerkamp, Claudia. "Ärzte und Professionalisierung in Deutschland: Überlegungen zum Wandel des Arztberufs in 19. Jahrhundert." *Geschichte und Gesellschaft* 6 (1980): 349–382.

Hull, David L. *Darwin and his Critics: The Reception of Darwin's Theory of Evolution by the Scientific Community.* Cambridge, Mass.: Harvard University Press, 1973.

Jeggle, Utz. "Alkohol und Industrialisierung." In *Rausch—Ekstase—Mystik. Grenzformen religiösen Erfahrung.* Düsseldorf: Patmos, 1978.

Jeschal, Godwin. *Politik und Wissenschaft deutscher Ärzte im Ersten Weltkrieg. Eine Untersuchung anhand der Fach- und Standespresse und der Protokolle des Reichstags.* Würzburger medizinhistorische Forschungen, Bd. 13. Pattensen: Horst Wellm, 1977.

Kelly, Alfred. *The Descent of Darwin: The Popularization of Darwinism in Germany, 1860–1914.* Chapel Hill: University of North Carolina Press, 1981.

Kevles, Daniel J. *In the Name of Eugenics: Genetics and the Uses of Human Heredity.* New York: Alfred A. Knopf, 1985.

Klass, Gert von. *Krupps: The Story of an Industrial Empire.* Trans. James Cleugh. London: Sidgwick and Jackson, 1954.

Klee, Ernst. "Euthanasie" im NS-Staat. Die "Vernichtung lebensunwerten Lebens." Frankfurt am Main: S. Fischer, 1983.

Knemeyer, Franz-Ludwig. "Polizei." *Economy and Society* 9 (1980): 172–196.

Knodel, John E. *The Decline of Fertility in Germany 1871–1939.* Princeton: Princeton University Press, 1974.

Kocka, Jürgen. "Industrielles Management: Konzeptionen und Modelle in Deutschland vor 1914." *Vierteljahsschrift für Sozial- und Wirtschaftsgeschichte* 56 (1969):332–372.

Köllmann, Wolfgang. "The Process of Urbanization in Germany at the Height of the Industrialization Period." *Journal of Contemporary History* 4 (1969):59–76.

Kotowski, Georg; Pöls, Werner; and Ritter, Gerhard A., eds. *Das wilhelminische Deutschland.* Frankfurt and Hamburg: Fischer, 1965.

Kraepelin, Emil. *One Hundred Years of Psychiatry.* Trans. Wade Barkin. New York: Citadel, 1962.

Kröner, Hans-Peter. "Die Eugenik in Deutschland von 1891 bis 1934." Med. diss., Münster, 1980.

Kroll, Jürgen. *Zur Entstehung und Institutionalisierung einer naturwissenschaftlichen und sozialpolitischen Bewegung: Die Entwicklung der Eugenik/Rassenhygiene bis zum Jahre 1933.* Sozialwiss. diss., Tübingen, 1983. Tübingen: privately printed.

Kudlien, Fridolf, ed. *Ärzte im Nationalsozialismus.* Cologne: Kiepenheuer & Witsch, 1985.

———. "Max v. Gruber und die frühe Hitlerbewegung." *Medizinhistorisches Journal* 17 (1982):373–389.

Lenz, Fritz. "Die soziologische Bedeutung der Selektion." In *Hundert Jahre Evolutionsforschung: Das wissenschaftliche Vermächtnis Charles Darwins,* ed. Gerhard Heberer, 368–396. Stuttgart: Gustav Fischer, 1960.

Ledbetter, Rosanna. *A History of the Malthusian League 1877–1927.* Columbus: Ohio State University Press, 1976.

Lilienthal, Georg. *Der "Lebensborn e.V.": Ein Instrument nationalsozialistischer Rassenpolitik.* Forschungen zur neueren Medizin- und Biologiegeschichte, Bd. 1. Stuttgart and New York: Gustav Fischer, 1985.

———. "Rassenhygiene im Dritten Reich. Krise und Wende." *Medizinhistorisches Journal* 14 (1979):114–133.

Lidtke, Vernon L. *The Outlawed Party: Social Democracy in Germany, 1878–1890.* Princeton: Princeton University Press, 1966.

Lowe, R. A. "Eugenicists, Doctors, and the Quest for National Efficiency: An Educational Crusade, 1900–1939." *History of Education* 8 (1979):293–306.

Ludmerer, Kenneth. "American Geneticists and the Eugenics Movement: 1905–35." *Journal of the History of Biology* 2 (1969):337–362.

———. *Genetics and American Society: An Historical Approach.* Baltimore: Johns Hopkins University Press, 1972.

Lutzhöft, Hans-Jürgen. *Der Nordische Gedanke in Deutschland 1920 bis 1940.* Kieler Historische Studien, Bd. 14. Stuttgart: Klett-Cotta, 1981.

MacKenzie, Donald. "Karl Pearson and the Professional Middle Class." *Annals of Science* 36 (1979):125–143.

———. "Eugenics in Britain." *Social Studies of Science* 6 (1976):499–532.

Manchester, William. *The Arms of Krupp.* Boston: Little, Brown and Co., 1968.

Mandelbaum, Maurice. *History, Man, and Reason: A Study in Nineteenth Century Thought.* Baltimore: The Johns Hopkins University Press, 1971.

Mann, Gunter. "Biologie und Geschichte: Ansätze und Versuche zur biologischen Theorie der Geschichte im 19. und beginnenden 20. Jahrhundert." *Medizinhistorisches Journal* 10 (1975):281–306.

――――. "Biologie und der 'neue Mensch.'" In *Medizin, Naturwissenschaft, Technik und das zweite Kaiserreich,* eds. Gunter Mann and Rolf Winau, 172–188. Göttingen: Vandenhoeck und Ruprecht, 1977.

――――. "Medizinisch-biologische Ideen und Modelle in der Gesellschaftslehre des 19. Jahrhunderts." *Medizinhistorisches Journal* 4 (1969):1–23.

――――. "Neue Wissenschaft im Rezeptionsbereich des Darwinismus: Eugenik—Rassenhygiene." *Berichte zur Wissenschaftsgeschichte* 1 (1978):101–111.

――――. "Rassenhygiene—Sozialdarwinismus." In *Biologismus im 19. Jahrhundert in Deutschland. Vorträge eines Symposiums vom 30. bis 31.10.1970 in Frankfurt am Main,* ed. Gunter Mann. Stuttgart: Ferdinand Enke, 1973.

――――. "Sozialbiologie auf dem Wege zur unmenschlichen Medizin des Dritten Reiches." In *Unmenschliche Medizin. Geschichtliche Erfahrungen, gegenwärtige Probleme und Ausblick auf die zukünftige Entwicklung. Seminar.* Bad Nauheimer Gespräche der Landesärztekammer Hessen. Mainz: Kirchheim, 1983.

Mazumdar, Pauline M. H. "The Eugenists and the Residuum: The Problem of the Urban Poor." *Bulletin of the History of Medicine* 54 (1980):204–215.

McHale, Victor E. and Johnson, Eric A. "Urbanization, Industrialization and Crime in Imperial Germany." *Social Science History* 1 (1976–1977):45–78, 210–247.

Mitschelich, Alexander, and Mielke, Fred, eds. *Medizin ohne Menschlichkeit: Dokumente des Nürnberger Ärzteprozesses.* Frankfurt am Main: S. Fischer, 1978.

Mock, Wolfgang. "'Manipulation von oben' oder Selbstorganisation an der Basis? Einige neuere Ansätze in der englischen Historiographie zur Geschichte des deutschen Kaiserreichs." *Historische Zeitschrift* 232 (1981):358–375.

Montagu, Ashley. *Man's Most Dangerous Myth: The Fallacy of Race.* 5th ed. Oxford: Oxford University Press, 1974.

Mosse, George L. *The Crisis of German Ideology: Intellectual Origins of the Third Reich.* New York: Grosset and Dunlap, 1964.

――――. *Toward the Final Solution: A History of European Racism.* London: J. M. Dent and Sons, 1978.

Mühlen, Patrik von zur. *Rassenideologien: Geschichte und Hintergründe.* Berlin and Bad Godesberg: J. H. W. Dietz, 1977.

Mühlmann, Wilhelm E. *Geschichte der Anthropologie.* 2d ed. Frankfurt am Main: Athenäum, 1968.

Müller, Joachim. "Sterilisation und Gesetzgebung bis 1933." Unpub. paper delivered at the Institut für die Geschichte der Medizin in Mainz, 7 November 1978.

Müller-Hegemann, Dietrich. "Über den Einfluß der Eugenik auf die deutsche Medizin." *Deutsche Gesundheitswesen* 14 (1959):429–436.

Müller-Hill, Benno. *Tödliche Wissenschaft: Die Aussonderung von Juden, Zigeunern und Geisteskranken 1933–1945.* Hamburg: Rowohlt, 1984.

Müssiggang, Albert. *Die soziale Frage in der historischen Schule der deutschen Nationalökonomie.* Tübingen: J. C. B. Mohr, 1968.

Muhlen, Norbert. *The Incredible Krupps. The Rise, Fall, and Comeback of Germany's Industrial Family.* New York: Henry Holt and Co., 1959.

Muncy, Lysbeth W. *The Junker in the Prussian Administration, 1888–1914.* New York: Howard Fertig, 1970.

Nagel, Günter. *Georges Vacher de Lapouge (1854–1936): Ein Beitrag zur Geschichte des Sozialdarwinismus in Frankreich.* Freiburger Forschungen zur Medizingeschichte. Freiburg i. B.: Hans Ferdinand Schulz, 1975.

Neumann, R. P. "The Sexual Question and the Social Democracy in Germany." *Journal of Social History* 7 (1974):271–286.

Nowak, Kurt. *"Euthanasie" und Sterilisierung im Dritten Reich. Die Konfrontation der evangelischen und katholischen Kirche mit dem "Gesetz zur Verhütung erbkranken Nachwuchses" und der "Euthanasie"-Aktion.* 3d ed. Göttingen: Vandenhoeck und Ruprecht, 1984.

Nye, Robert A. "Heredity or Milieu: The Foundations of Modern European Criminological Theory." *Isis* 67 (1976):335–355.

Pickens, Donald K. *Eugenics and the Progressives.* Nashville, Tenn.: Vanderbilt University Press, 1968.

Platen-Hallermund, Alice. *Die Tötung Geisteskranken in Deutschland.* Frankfurt am Main: Frankfurter Hefte, 1948.

Poliakov, Leon. *Der arische Mythos: Zu den Quellen von Rassismus und Nationalismus.* Trans. Margarete Vehjakob. Vienna: Europa, 1977.

Proctor, Robert N. "Pawns or Pioneers? The Role of Doctors in the Origins of Nazi Racial Science." Unpub. Ms., Harvard University, 1982.

Projektgruppe "Volk und Gesundheit," ed. *Volk und Gesundheit. Heilen und Vernichten im Nationalsozialismus.* Tübingen: Tübinger Vereinigung für Volkskunde, 1982.

Querner, Hans. "Darwin, sein Werk und der Darwinismus." In *Biologismus im 19. Jahrhundert in Deutschland*, ed. Gunter Mann. Stuttgart: Ferdinand Enke, 1973.

————. "Ideologisch-weltanschauliche Konsequenten der Lehre Darwins." *Studium Generale* 24 (1971):231–245.

Raeff, Marc. "The Well-Ordered Police State and the Development of Modernity in Seventeenth and Eighteenth Century Europe: An Attempt at a Comparative Approach." *American Historical Review* 80 (1975):1221–1243.

Rehse, Helga. "Euthanasie, Vernichtung unwerten Lebens und Rassenhygiene in Programmschriften vor dem Ersten Weltkrieg." Med. diss., Heidelberg, 1969.

Ringer, Fritz. *The Decline of the German Mandarins: The German Academic Community, 1890–1933.* Cambridge, Mass.: Harvard University Press, 1969.

Roberts, James S. "Der Alkoholkonsum deutscher Arbeiter im 19. Jahrhundert." *Geschichte und Gesellschaft* 6 (1980):220–242.

————. *Drink, Temperance and the Working Class in Nineteenth Century Germany.* Boston: Allen & Unwin, 1984.

Rose, Nikolas. "The Psychological Complex: Mental Measurement and Social Administration." *Ideology and Consciousness* 5 (1979):5–68.

Rosen, George. *A History of Public Health.* New York: MD Publications, 1958.

Rosenberg, Charles. *No Other Gods: On Science and American Social Thought.* Baltimore: The Johns Hopkins University Press, 1976.

Rosenberg, Hans. "Wirtschaftskonjunktur, Gesellschaft und Politik." In *Moderne deutsche Sozialgeschichte*, ed. Hans-Ulrich Wehler, 225–253. Cologne: Kiepenheuer und Witsch, 1976.

Rubenstein, Richard L. *The Cunning of History: The Holocaust and the American Future.* New York: Harper & Row, 1975.

Roth, Guenther. *The Social Democrats in Imperial Germany.* 1963. Reprint. New York: Arno, 1979.

Saller, Karl. *Die Rassenlehre des Nationalsozialismus in Wissenschaft und Propaganda.* Darmstadt: Progress, 1961.

Schipperges, Heinrich. *Utopien der Medizin: Geschichte und Kritik der ärztlichen Ideologie des 19. Jahrhunderts.* Salzburg: Otto Müller, 1968.

Schlach, Joachim. "Die Kruppsiedlungen—Wohnungsbau im Interesse eines Industriekonzerns." In *Kapitalistischer Städtebau*, ed. Hans Helms and Jörn Janssen. Neuwied and Berlin: Hermann Luchterhand, 1971.

Schneider, William. "Toward the Improvement of the Human Race: The History of Eugenics in France." *Journal of Modern History* 54 (1982): 268–291.

————. "Eugenics in France." *New Perspectives on the History of Eugenics,* ed. Mark B. Adams. New York: Oxford University Press, forthcoming.

Schraepler, Ernst, ed. *Quellen zur Geschichte der sozialen Frage in Deutschland.* Quellensammlung zur Kulturgeschichte, Bd. 9. 2d ed. Göttingen: Musterschmidt, 1964.

Searle, Geoffrey R. *Eugenics and Politics in Britain 1900–1914.* Science in History, 3. Leyden: Noordhoff International, 1976.

————. "Eugenics and Politics in Britain in the 1930s." *Annals of Science* 36 (1979):159–169.

————. *The Quest for National Efficiency. A Study in British Politics and Political Thought 1899–1914.* Oxford: Blackwell, 1971.

Seidelmann, William E. "From Hippocrates to the Holocaust: Genetics and Genocide." Unpub. paper delivered at McMaster University, Hamilton, Ontario, Canada, 14 February 1985.

Seidler, Eduard. "Evolutionismus in Frankreich." *Sudhoffs Archiv* 53 (1969):362–377.

————. "Der politische Standort des Arztes im zweiten Kaiserreich." In *Medizin, Naturwissenschaft, Technik und das zweite Kaiserreich,* eds. Gunter Mann and Rolf Winau, 87–102. Göttingen: Vandenhoeck und Ruprecht, 1977.

————, and Nagel, Günter. "Georges Vacher de Lapouge (1854–1936) und der Sozialdarwinismus in Frankreich." In *Biologismus im 19. Jahrhundert in Deutschland,* ed. Gunter Mann. Stuttgart: Ferdinand Enke, 1973.

Semmel, Bernard. *Imperialism and Social Reform.* New York: Anchor, 1968.

Soloway, Richard A. "Neo-Malthusians, Eugenists, and the Declining Birth Rate in England, 1900–1918." *Albion* 10 (1978):264–286.

————. "Counting the Degenerates: The Statistics of Race Deterioration in Edwardian England." *Journal of Contemporary History* 17 (1982): 137–164.

Stark, Gary. *Entrepreneurs of Ideology: Neoconservative Publishers in Germany, 1890–1933.* Chapel Hill: University of North Carolina Press, 1981.

Steinberg, Hans-Josef. *Sozialismus und deutsche Sozialdemokratie.* Bonn-Bad Godesberg: J. H. W. Dietz, 1976.

Stepan, Nancy Leys. "Eugenics in Brazil, 1917–1940." In *New Perspectives on the History of Eugenics,* ed. Mark B. Adams. New York: Oxford University Press, forthcoming.

Stern, Fritz. *The Failure of Illiberalism: Essays on the Political Culture of Modern Germany.* Chicago: University of Chicago Press, 1975.

Steiner, Andreas. *Das nervöse Zeitalter: Der Begriff der Nervosität bei Laien und Ärzten in Deutschland und Österreich um 1900.* Zürcher medizingeschichtliche Abhandlungen, no. 21. Zurich: Juris, 1964.

Stürmer, Michael, ed. *Das kaiserliche Deutschland.* Düsseldorf: Droste, 1970.

Sturtevant, A. H. *A History of Genetics.* New York: Harper and Row, 1965.

Thomann, Klaus-Dieter. "Auf dem Weg in den Faschismus: Medizin in Deutschland von der Jahrhundertwende bis 1933." In *Medizin, Faschismus und Widerstand. Drei Beitrage.* Cologne: Pahl-Rugenstein, 1985.

————. "Die Zusammenarbeit der Sozialhygieniker Alfred Grotjahn und Alfons Fischer." *Medizinhistorisches Journal* 14 (1979):251–274.

Thompson, Larry V. "*Lebensborn* and the Eugenics Policy of the *Reichsführer-SS.*" *Central European History* 4 (1971):57–71.

Vondung, Klaus, ed. *Das wilhelminische Bildungsbürgertum: Zur Sozialgeschichte seiner Ideen.* Göttingen: Vandenhoeck und Ruprecht, 1976.

Waldinger, Robert J. "The High Priests of Nature: Medicine in Germany, 1883–1933." B. A. thesis, Harvard University, 1973.

Walker, Mack. *German Home Towns: Community, State, and General Estate 1648–1871.* Ithaca: Cornell University Press, 1971.

Walser, Hans, ed. *August Forel: Briefe—Correspondenz 1864–1927.* Bern: Hans Huber, 1968.

Walter, Richard D. "What Became of the Degenerate. A Brief History of a Concept." *Journal of the History of Medicine* (1956):422–429.

Weber, Max. *Weber: Selections in Translation.* Ed. W. G. Runciman. Trans. Eric Mathews. Cambridge: Cambridge University Press, 1978.

Wehler, Hans-Ulrich. *Das Deutsche Kaiserreich 1871–1918.* Göttingen: Vandenhoeck und Ruprecht, 1977.

————. "Sozialdarwinismus im expandierenden Industriestaat." In *Deutschland in der Weltpolitik des 19. und 20. Jahrhunderts. Festschrift für Fritz Fischer.* Düsseldorf: Bertelsmann, 1973.

Weindling, Paul. "The Medical Profession, Social Hygiene and the Birth Rate in Germany, 1914–1918." Unpublished Ms., 1983.

————. "Die Preußische Medizinalverwaltung und die 'Rassenhygiene.'"

Anmerkungen zur Gesundheitspolitik der Jahre 1905–1933."
Zeitschrift für Sozialreform 30 (1984):675–687.

———. "Race, Blood and Politics." *The Times Higher Education Supplement,* 19 July 1985, 13.

———. "Soziale Hygiene: Eugenik und medizinische Praxis—Der Fall Alfred Grotjahn." *Das Argument: Jahrbuch für kritische Medizin* (1984):6–20.

———. "Theories of the Cell State in Imperial Germany." In *Biology, Medicine and Society 1840–1940,* ed. Charles Webster, 99–155. Cambridge: Cambridge University Press, 1981.

———. "Weimar Eugenics: The Kaiser Wilhelm Institute for Anthropology, Human Heredity and Eugenics in Social Context." *Annals of Science* 42 (1985):303–318.

Weiss, Sheila F. "Wilhelm Schallmayer and the Logic of German Eugenics." *Isis* 77 (1986):33–46.

———. "Race Hygiene and the Rational Management of National Efficiency: Wilhelm Schallmayer and the Origins of German Eugenics, 1890–1920." Ph.D. diss., The Johns Hopkins University, 1983.

———. "The Race Hygiene Movement in Germany." Forthcoming in *Osiris* 3 (1987).

Wendel, Günter. *Der Kaiser-Wilhelm-Gesellschaft 1911–1914.* Berlin-East: Akademie, 1975.

Wertham, Frederic. *A Sign For Cain.* New York: Warner Paperback Library, 1973.

Wettley, Annemarie. "Entartung und Erbsünde: Der Einfluß des medizinischen Entartungsbegriffs auf den literarischen Naturalismus." *Hochland* 51 (1958–1959):348–358.

———. "Der Entartungsbegriff und seine geistigen Abzweigungen in der Psychopathologie des 19. und 20. Jahrhunderts." *Jahrbuch für Psychologie* 6 (1958–1959):279–285.

———. *Von der "Psychopathia Sexualis" zur Sexualwissenschaft.* Beiträge zur Sexualforschung, no. 17. Stuttgart: Ferdinand Enke, 1959.

———. "Zur Problemgeschichte der dégénérescence." *Sudhoffs Archiv* 43 (1959):193–212.

Wuttke-Groneberg, Walter, ed. *Medizin im Nationalsozialismus. Ein Arbeitsbuch.* 2d ed. Rottenburg: Schwäbische Verlagsgesellschaft, 1982.

Yeboa, Joseph. "Zum sozialen und eugenischen Darwinismus am Ausgang des 19. Jahrhunderts." Med. diss., Heidelberg, 1968.

Young, E. J. *Gobineau und der Rassismus: Eine Kritik der anthropologischen Geschichtstheorie.* Meisenheim am Glan: Anton Hain, 1968.

Young, Robert M. "Darwin's Metaphor: Does Nature Select?" *Monist* 55 (1971):442–503.

———. "Evolutionary Biology and Ideology Then and Now." *Social Studies of Science* 1 (1971):177–206.

———. "The Historiographic and Ideological Contexts of the Nineteenth-Century Debate on Man's Place in Nature." In *Changing Perspectives in the History of Science: Essays in Honour of Joseph Needham*, ed. M. Teich and R. Young, 344–438. London: Hanemann, 1973.

———. "Malthus and the Evolutionists: The Common Context of Biological and Social Theory." *Past and Present*, no. 43 (1969):109–145.

Zmarzlik, Hans G. "Sozialdarwinismus in Deutschland als geschichtliches Problem." *Vierteljahreshefte für Zeitgeschichte* 11 (1963):246–273.

INDEX

Designer: U.C. Press Staff
Compositor: Andresen Typographers
Text: 10/13 Palatino
Display: 18/20 Palatino